Occupational Therapist Registered OTR®
Certification Examination

Official NBCOT Study Guide

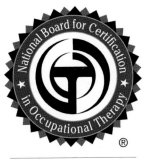

Serving the Public Interest

National Board for Certification in Occupational Therapy, Inc.
12 South Summit Avenue, Suite 100
Gaithersburg, MD 20877-4150

www.nbcot.org

Our Mission...

Above all else, the mission of the National Board for Certification in Occupational Therapy, Inc. (NBCOT®) is to serve the public interest. We provide a world-class standard for certification of occupational therapy practitioners. NBCOT will develop, administer, and continually review a certification process based on current and valid standards that provide reliable indicators of competence for the practice of occupational therapy.

National Board for Certification in Occupational Therapy, Inc.
12 South Summit Avenue, Suite 100
Gaithersburg, MD 20877-4150
http://www.nbcot.org

Printed in the United States of America.

ISBN 0-9785178-3-0

The National Board for Certification in Occupational Therapy, Inc. (NBCOT®) is pleased to publish the Official Examination Study Guide for the OCCUPATIONAL THERAPY REGISTERED OTR® (OTR) Certification Examination. The occupational therapy content of this guide has been aligned to the examination test specifications of NBCOT's 2007 Practice Analysis Study. The results of this study were used to guide examination items that will subsequently be used on NBCOT certification examinations beginning January 2009.

The purpose of this study guide is to provide:

- a tool that will assist candidates gain an understanding of the certification process;
- examples of practice-focused sample items for the OTR; and
- a means to assist candidates with their test preparation.

The primary purpose for developing this study guide is to provide information to candidates that can be used to support and augment their overall examination preparation activities. By purchasing this guide, no inference should be made or assumed that by using this guide it ensures success on the certification examination.

The development of this guide, and most importantly the certification examination, would not have been possible without the professionalism and expertise of a dedicated legion of OTR practitioners and educators who participated in NBCOT's item writing activities and/or on the Certification Examination Validation Committee (CEVC). The breadth and depth of the material in this guide would not have been possible without their participation.

Paul Grace, MS, CAE
President and Chief Executive Officer, NBCOT

NBCOT... serving the public interest

Contents

Historically, regulation of the health professions in the United States began with a necessity to protect the public from the under-educated and under-trained professional. Over time, licensure, credentialing and certification have continued the tradition of protecting the public but have also increased their scope of activity to continuously improve the quality of practice in the profession.

Certification is a process by which key required competencies for practice are measured, and the professional is endorsed by a board of his/her peers (Barnhart, 1997). Earned certification means an individual has met a specified quality standard that reflects nationally-accepted practice principles and values (McClain, Richardson & Wyatt, 2004). The purpose of awarding the credential – OCCUPATIONAL THERAPIST REGISTERED (OTR®) - is to identify for the public those persons who have demonstrated the knowledge and the skills necessary to provide occupational therapy services. Certification has become the hallmark credential for professionals in a variety of industries, often serving as a benchmark for hiring and promotion (Microsoft, 2003). For more than 70 years, the OTR "mark" has been recognized by agencies, employers, payers, and consumers as viable symbols of quality educated and currently prepared practitioners.

The National Board for Certification in Occupational Therapy, Inc. (NBCOT®) is a not-for-profit credentialing agency responsible for the development and implementation of policies related to the certification of occupational therapy practitioners in the United States. This independent national credentialing agency grants the OTR certification to eligible individuals. The primary mission of NBCOT is to "serve the public interest." NBCOT certification uses a formal process to grant a certification credential to an individual who: 1) meets academic and practice experience requirements; 2) successfully completes a comprehensive examination to assess knowledge and skills for practice; and 3) agrees to adhere to the NBCOT Candidate/ Certificant Code of Conduct. Currently, 50 states, Guam, Puerto Rico and the District of Columbia require NBCOT initial certification for occupational therapy state regulation, e.g., licensing.

Overview and Purpose of the Study Guide

This study guide has six sections:

- Section 1 contains information about adult learning including thinking critically, learning as an adult, scheduling time for study, and controlling the study environment.

- Section 2 examines strategies for developing successful study habits such as using memory effectively, avoiding procrastination, and utilizing cooperative learning techniques.

- Section 3 considers general test-taking strategies including things to do before, during, and after the test, overcoming test anxiety, and guidelines for answering multiple-choice questions.

- Section 4 refers specifically to the NBCOT certification examination, including how NBCOT uses the results of practice analysis studies to guide test construction, and general administrative procedures specific to the NBCOT certification examination.

- Section 5 contains 100 multiple-choice OTR sample items representative of the domains and task areas found in the test blueprint. Although the items included in the study guide practice test are grouped by domain and task areas to illustrate the type of questions that may be representative of a particular domain, questions on the actual certification examination will not appear grouped by domain, but will be randomized. None of the questions included in this study guide will appear on the NBCOT certification examination. In addition to presenting sample items, this section also contains an answer key, a rationale for the correct response, an explanation of why the distractors are incorrect, and references for additional information.

- Section 6 contains ten (10) sample scenario-related items spanning a range of populations and practice settings. In addition to presenting sample scenarios, this section also contains an answer key, a rationale for the correct response, and explanation of why the distractors are incorrect, and references for additional information.

- Appendix A contains a copy of the OTR Examination Readiness Tool, Appendix B includes a reference list, Appendix C provides a listing of standard abbreviations used on the certification examination, Appendix D includes interventions, service components, and settings commonly used on the certification examination, and Appendix E includes the 2007 Blueprint Specifications for the OTR validated domain, task, and knowledge statements.

This study guide should be used as only one tool in preparing to take the certification examination. The examination questions are designed to test the knowledge necessary for entry-level practice. Reviewing course materials, texts, and fieldwork experiences are other ways that candidates can prepare for the certification examination. This study guide will supplement preparation efforts by providing information on the testing process and the structure of the questions that are used on the NBCOT certification examination.

NBCOT does not administer, approve, or endorse review or preparatory courses for the certification examination. It is NBCOT's mission that the OTR certification examination is reflective of current entry-level occupational therapy practice. Practice tests, available on NBCOT's website at *www.nbcot.org*, provide additional opportunities for test preparation. Certification examination review courses are advertised and available to candidates. However, these courses are not endorsed by NBCOT.

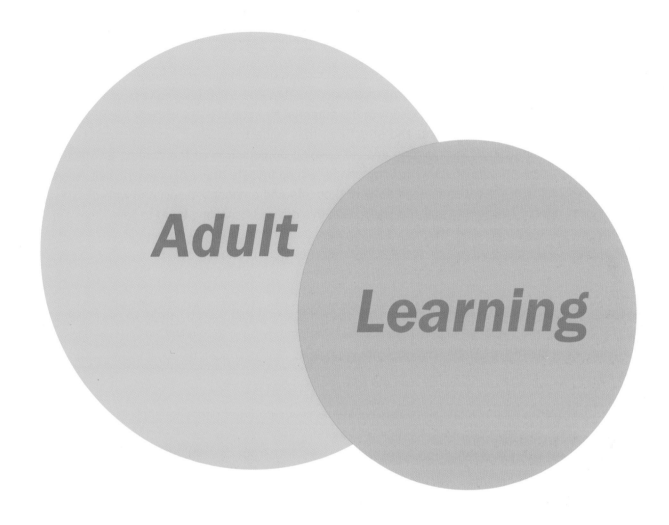

Thinking Critically

Learning to think critically is one of the most significant activities of adult life (Brookfield, 1987). Indeed, it can be argued that without critical thinking, the individual views the world through a single, isolated lens, with no awareness of how others view their actions, or respect for the way others behave or make decisions about their world. To think critically is to become open to alternative ways of looking at, and behaving in, the world. As Brookfield (1987) reminds us, it is through critical thinking that we learn to pay attention to the context in which we (and others) think, act, and behave.

Critical thinking should be a core skill for all successful occupational therapy practitioners. It is through critical thinking that the occupational therapy practitioner creates and recreates aspects of the client's life. Critical thinkers are innovators, concerned with the potential for improvement while at the same time, respecting diversity of values, behaviors, and structures that guide the client's world. Critical thinking entails continual questioning of assumptions and an ongoing appreciation of the context in which life occurs. For example, the occupational therapy practitioner will appreciate that a person who has recently become a wheelchair user will experience an array of thoughts and emotions associated with this newly acquired mobility device. The person may feel happy that this device is enabling them to gain access into their community. On the other hand, they may feel embarrassed, or frustrated for others to see that they are having to rely on a mobility device to do the things that they were previously able to do.

All occupational therapy entry-level curricula seek to develop critical thinking skills to prepare their students for successful future practice. However, the skill of critical thinking can also be used as an important strategy for studying and preparing to take high stakes examinations such as the NBCOT OTR certification examination. The following provides a framework of how to apply critical thinking to your studying routines:

1. *Define what it is that you want to learn.* You may be familiar with the anatomical implications of ulnar nerve palsy for example, but want to know more about how this impacts thumb mobility and the challenges posed by this condition for a homemaker caring for a young child. In this sense, you could use critical thinking to help you appreciate the perspective of this homemaker. Define your learning into simple phrases such as:

    - How does the impairment affect ability to button the baby's clothes?
    - How might this impact ability to carry out grooming tasks?
    - Would adaptations be needed to open packets of formula?

2. *Think about what you already know about the subject.* Critical thinking will help you to identify strengths and gaps in your knowledge. Tapping into your previous experiences from fieldwork, labs, case studies, and readings, will give you a foundation upon which to build your learning. It will also help you to identify any prejudices that may be coloring the way you are currently conducting your studying. For example, you may be reluctant to invest much time in considering how you might design a pre-vocational skills program for someone with a substance abuse disorder if you have an underlying prejudice about people who abuse alcohol. Addressing these prejudices will enable you to view situations with an open mind, and aid your studying and ongoing journey towards successful future practice.

3. *Identify resources.* Critical thinking is about recognizing and using all the resources that are available to you. In this sense, consider resources in the widest possible context, have an open mind. These are a few you may consider, expand on these and design your own list:

   ▣ People – professors, fieldwork educators, mentors, peer group, community members, case studies
   ▣ Materials – textbooks, journal readings, reflective journals, class notes, lab exercises, videos or DVDs
   ▣ Environments – fieldwork, community facilities, specialist clinics, adaptive workplaces, inpatient services

4. *Ask questions.* Use your critical thinking skills to enhance your understanding. Do you hold underlying beliefs about this disorder and is this influencing your studying? Does this author have prejudices about the information they are presenting? Is this professor telling you the full story about what it is like living with this disability? Continue to ask questions – why/what/how/if...

5. *Organize the information you have gathered.* Use your critical thinking skills to examine patterns and make connections across your learning. For example, you have reviewed your understanding about ulnar nerve palsy, talked to an occupational therapy practitioner who has treated people who have this condition, discussed ways this condition may affect household occupations with your peers, and identified possible short-term and long-term treatment goals from key texts.

6. *Demonstrate your knowledge.* Pulling all this information together, think of ways to demonstrate what you now know. Use lists, flowcharts, and summary statements to highlight key information. Discuss comparisons and similarities of disorders and strategies for overcoming occupational challenges. Write up an assessment report with recommendations for therapy.

> *Remember, have an open mind to enable you to gather resources to aid your learning. Group information together to increase understanding. Use critical thinking skills to enhance your studying.*

Learning as an Adult

Through your occupational therapy education, you will have identified that there are many different ways to learn information. You will also be familiar with evaluating and selecting the most appropriate learning strategy to meet the needs of the clients you are working with. You can use the same strategies to help you identify the best ways for *you* to learn information in order to help you study for the certification examination.

As an adult learner who has engaged in a comprehensive program of study to prepare for a career in occupational therapy, you will recognize that these are some of the ways you have most likely approached your learning:

   ▣ Taken a self-directed approach
   ▣ Drawn upon a reservoir of life experiences that serve as a resource for your studying
   ▣ Driven by a need to know, do, or find out something new
   ▣ Utilized problem-centered, or creative problem-solving strategies to trigger learning experiences
   ▣ Been intrinsically motivated to learn as a way to reaching your goal to become an occupational therapy practitioner

It is not unusual however, particularly during transition stages (like preparing to take the certification examination!), for learners to question and re-evaluate their motivation for learning. If you take an adult learning approach to these questions and re-evaluations, it will help you to tap into previous strategies for effective learning, and hopefully assist you with renewing your motivation for study.

The following is a list of helpful strategies that reflect adult learning principles:

1. *Take an active role in planning your studying by setting realistic study goals and expected time commitments.*

2. *Evaluate your progress.* Check off your study goals regularly, demonstrate your knowledge, continually question, and reward yourself for a job well done.

3. *Be open to new experiences – people, resources, materials, and environments.* Think outside of the box, who or what could help you learn more about what it is like to have this disability?

4. *Recognize the value of past experiences.* Recall experiences from your fieldwork, group discussions, and creative projects. Make connections between these and new learning opportunities.

5. *Develop an awareness of what helps you learn best.* Exploit these methods. For example, you may recognize that being able to discuss information in a group helps you to assimilate information. From this, you organize a weekly study group that focuses on preparing to take the certification examination.

6. *Don't be afraid to ask for help.* Academic counseling centers, learning centers, writing centers, reading and/or study skills centers, and student service centers, are just a few resources available to students studying in professional academic programs. Adult learning embraces the notion that it is appropriate to ask for guidance to assist with the learning experience.

> *Remember, being an adult learner means taking responsibility for your learning. Set goals, evaluate, monitor, adapt, develop awareness of past and new experiences, and use resources wisely.*

Scheduling Time for Studying

A common student complaint is that there is not enough time to go around. The time pressures involved in being an adult learner pursuing an occupational therapy education is enormous. Not only does the student typically face tightly scheduled classes, he or she is also expected to carry out several hours of preparation for each hour spent in the classroom, along with studying for tests and writing assignments. This, along with fieldwork and other community-based learning activities, soon add up to a full-time occupation. Many students in an entry-level occupational therapy program find that they have additional commitments related to part-time working and family/social responsibilities taking up even more of their time each week.

The way a student uses time, or wastes time, is largely a matter of habit patterns. By the time a student is ready to graduate from an occupational therapy program and start preparing to study for the certification examination, these study habits will be well developed. Inefficient study habits can be changed however, and it is worth reviewing strategies for time scheduling here, reinforcing adult learning principles of taking responsibility for managing time when studying for the certification examination.

1. *Plan enough time for study.* Review the way you have planned your time to prepare for key assignments during your occupational therapy education. Think of occasions when you achieved a particularly successful grade or outcome, assess the factors that contributed to this including the amount of time you dedicated for preparation. In terms of the preparation you covered, knowledge that was being tested, and type of test/assignment given, estimate in hours/days how much preparation you carried out for this test. Now compare this to the certification examination. What are the similarities and differences between the two tests/assignments? Begin to formulate how much time you will need to optimally study for the certification examination. You are your own best estimator, you know how you work, and how much time you will need to prepare and plan for a successful study schedule. Be honest and realistic with your estimation.

2. *Study at the same time each day.* To develop effective study habits, or modify inefficient study routines, it is recommended that students schedule certain hours that are used for studying throughout the day, every day. This enables a habitual, systematic, study routine to develop and helps to maintain an active approach to learning and preparing for the test.

3. *Make use of free time.* There are many opportunities throughout the day when students could take advantage of additional study time. Carry around a small notebook with the lists, summary statements, and flowcharts you have developed from your studying of specific occupational therapy practice. Use time between classes, riding the bus, waiting for appointments, walking on the treadmill to review your notes. Tap into your critical thinking, question your notes, jot down alternative explanations.

4. *Schedule relaxation time.* Just as your occupational therapy training has emphasized the need for occupational balance, students should build in relaxation time into their study schedule. It is more efficient to study hard for a definite period of time, and then stop for a few minutes, than attempt to study on indefinitely. Plan for a 10-15 minute break after every 60-90 minutes of focused study. During this break time, ensure that you move away from your study materials, stretch, and use your other senses such as listening to music or drinking a glass of water, to give your mind a rest from the focused studying. Be disciplined however, to return to your study materials after each allocated break period.

5. *Review regularly.* On a weekly basis, review the progress you have made towards reaching your study goals. Are you still on schedule? Do you need to build in additional study time? Is there flexibility in your schedule to allow for unforeseen events? This review time should prompt you to acknowledge just how well you are doing and build your confidence in preparing to take the certification examination.

6. *Build in time for longer periods of occupational balance.* As well as taking short breaks between periods of focused study, plan for longer periods of "away time" when you can engage in enjoyable activities. Use these scheduled activities as a reward for reaching your study goals and as a way of nurturing your body before returning to your set study schedule.

Remember, as an adult learner, you can take responsibility for developing an effective study schedule, build in relaxation time, and be realistic with your time goals.

Controlling the Study Environment

As an adult learner, you not only need to take responsibility for scheduling time for studying, you need to take control of your study environment. Your occupational therapy training has emphasized the importance of considering the environment in which your clients perform their daily occupations. You can apply the same skill to meet your own needs when designing a study environment to enhance your preparations for taking the certification examination. The following is a list of such environmental strategies:

1. *Set aside a fixed place for study.* This ensures that over time, this place becomes associated with studying behavior, and it will be easier for you to engage in study activities.

2. *Identify factors that increase your ability to focus.* For some people this means making the room as quiet as possible, for others this means putting on some background music. Check if the room is a comfortable temperature, that you have sufficient drinks/snacks close at hand, that your phone is turned off, and that you have all the materials you will need for studying.

3. *Post the goal or goals associated for your planned study session next to your work desk.* This will help you to focus and be an effective motivational tool.

4. *Use symbols, or rituals, to get you in the studying frame of mind.* This might include wearing a particular article of clothing or jewelry, reading a special poem, looking at a favorite picture, or organizing your workspace. Whatever the action, the symbol/ritual will, over time, become associated with studying behavior.

5. *If your mind starts to wander, stand up and look away from your study materials.* Re-connect with the symbol/ritual you used at the start of your study session. Return refreshed and ready to refocus.

6. *Build in regular review periods.* Post times above your desk when you plan to stop and verbalize what it is you have been studying.

7. *Keep a reminder pad beside you while you study.* Use the pad to jot down thoughts if your mind begins to wander onto other activities besides your studying. Once you have written down the thought, return to your studying. This action will help you to re-focus, while at the same time, provide a reminder to you later of things you have to do.

> *Remember, as an adult learner, you can take control of your study environment. Identify factors that will enhance your study environment and put them into play.*

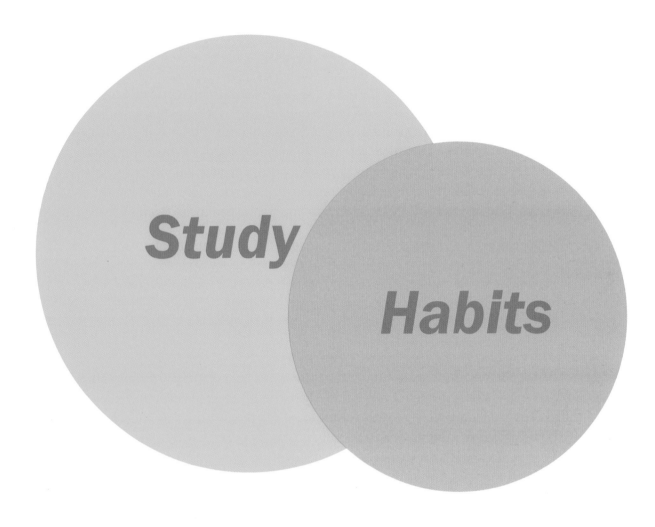

Study

Habits

$\mathcal{S}_{ection}$ I of this guide considered adult learning and encouraged the reader to use adult learning principles, such as critical thinking, as a way to organize and conduct studying for the certification examination. This, along with specific emphasis on taking responsibility for managing time and the study environment, provides a strong foundation on which to develop effective study habits. This next section gives an overview of specific study habits. While it is not intended to be an exhaustive list, the reader is encouraged to use the list as a trigger for examining their current study habits, and as a springboard for considering alternative study methods.

Effective Habits for Studying

(Adapted from Covey, S. R. (1989). *The 7 Habits of Highly Effective People.* New York: Simon & Schuster.)

- *Take responsibility for yourself.* Tapping into the principles outlined in the section on adult learning, remind yourself that in order to succeed, you need to make decisions about your priorities (What interventions do you need to study this week?), your time (How much time should I spend reviewing my knowledge on spinal cord levels?), and your resources (I need to coordinate my notes on major mood disorders with the case notes I gathered from my mental health fieldwork).

- *Center yourself around your needs.* Remind yourself, "What is important to me now?" The certification examination can be viewed as the ending of one journey (your academic preparation), and the gateway to your next journey (the start of your professional occupational therapy career). It should be a natural step in your progression towards your chosen career. Use these thoughts to motivate as you set up your study schedule.

- *Follow up on priorities.* Keep to your schedule as far as possible. If you have fallen behind, take steps to review your progress, highlight the reasons for falling behind (Did you set unrealistic study goals? Did you allow others to interrupt your studying?), and try and build in methods to overcome these difficulties in the future (review goals, revise to ensure they are manageable, tell others that you need some undisturbed study time).

- *Congratulate yourself regularly.* Remind yourself of the progress you have made to date – the classes, fieldwork, labs, assignments, and tests completed up to this point. Use your study schedule and completed study goals to highlight the progress you are making towards your goal of taking the certification examination.

- *Consider other solutions.* If you are having difficulty understanding readings from textbooks and class notes, think of alternative ways for you to make sense of this material. For example, you might consider talking it through with one of your professors, revisiting a fieldwork site, or joining a peer study group.

> *Remind yourself of the progress you have made to date. Use your study schedule and completed study tasks to highlight the progress you are making towards your goal.*

Concentrating When Studying

Just as we all have the ability to concentrate, there will be times when it is difficult for us to remain focused. Our mind may wander from one topic to another, worries about the consequences of not doing well on the test, allowing outside distractions to interfere with our study routine, and finding the material difficult or uninteresting can contribute to loss of concentration while trying to study. There are two effective methods for increasing ability to concentrate.

1. *Scheduled Worry Time.* Set aside a specific time each day to think about the things that keep entering your mind and interfere with your studying. When you become aware of a distracting thought, remind yourself that you have a special time to think about them. Let the thought go, and keep your appointment to worry or think about those distracting issues at the time you have scheduled for these. Let your mind return to focus on your immediate activity of studying.

2. *Be Here Now.* When you notice your thoughts wandering, say to yourself, "Be here now." Gently bring your attention back to where you want it to be – your notes on developmental milestones, for example. If your mind wanders again, repeat the phrase "Be here now." and gently bring your attention back. Continually practice this technique and you should notice that the period of time between your straying thoughts gets a little longer each time. Be patient and keep at it.

Using Memory Effectively

While acronyms (invented combination of letters), acrostic (invented sentence where first letter of each word is a cue to an idea you need to remember), rhyme-keys, and chaining are recognized techniques for recalling systems or lists of information (and they are described at length in many other generic study guide texts), they are perhaps not the most effective methods for studying and recalling material in preparation for NBCOT's certification examination. Test items on this examination rely on candidates demonstrating their knowledge as it applies to the practice of occupational therapy.

Alternative methods should include using memory of situations and experiences as applied to practice. For example, when studying the ulnar nerve, the candidate may associate actions of the flexor muscles with specific tasks such as holding a pencil or utensil. Fieldwork experiences may also act as a strong memory aid where candidates recall working with a particular individual who had a similar disability to the ones presented on the examination.

Using memory in this sense will enable you to apply your knowledge to the practice of occupational therapy.

Thinking Aloud

Through your learning about human development during your occupational therapy education, you are probably familiar with the term "private speech." Private speech is an accepted way for infants and children to think aloud or say what they are thinking as a way of demonstrating knowledge. Children use private speech to practice words, express ideas, form sentences, and as a way to make sense of their external world. Thinking aloud is essential to early learning. As we grow older, thinking aloud or private speech, becomes internalized. However, whenever we encounter unfamiliar or demanding activities in our adult lives, we can use private speech as a way to overcome obstacles and acquire new skills.

The more we engage our brain on multiple levels, the more we are able to make connections and retain what we learn. We can apply these same techniques to our study habits. As well as reading, we can create images, listen, talk with others, and talk with ourselves about the concepts we are learning. Some of us like to talk things through with someone else as a way of increasing our understanding, and others do not need another person around to talk with in this process. Using multiple senses and experiences to process and reinforce our learning is an individualized process, but one that can be very effective in helping to understand and retain knowledge.

> *Remember to engage your brain on multiple levels while studying. Utilize various techniques, senses and experiences to process and reinforce your learning.*

Avoiding Procrastination

Procrastination can stop you from achieving the study goals you wish to reach. Here are some ways to help overcome procrastination:

Ask yourself, "What is it that I want to do?"

- What is your final objective, the end result?
    I want to review my notes on occupational therapy frames of reference.

- What are the major steps to get there?
    I need to locate my class notes.
    I need to check out the theory book from the library.
    I need to access my fieldwork journal where I wrote a case study using 3 major frames of reference.
    I need to prepare a grid showing the major frames of reference for my study group.

- What have you done so far?
    I've got the book from the library.
    I've found my fieldwork journal.
    I've bought some large sheets of grid paper and marker pens.

Next ask yourself, "Why do I want to do this?"

- What is your biggest motivation?
    I want to have all the frames of reference clear in my mind.
    I'd like to apply theoretical concepts to practice application.
    I need to feel I am contributing to the study group.
    I want to feel prepared for the certification exam.

- What other positive results will flow from achieving this goal?
    I can talk about my knowledge during recruitment interviews.
    I can use them to aid my documentation when writing up treatment plans in the future.
    I can assist members in my study group to understand the similarities and differences between the theories.

List what stands in your way:

- What is in your power to change?

  If I chose to review a frame of reference that I'm interested in first, it will help me to feel motivated to study the others.

  I don't want to prepare this grid in case I mess it up, but if I draft it on the computer I can build it up gradually.

  There are so many to cover, I'll never get through them all. If I group them together into categories, they will be more manageable for me to study.

- What resources beside yourself do you need?

  I could use some help with drawing up this grid. I am going to ask one other member from the study group to work on this with me.

- What will happen if I don't progress?

  I won't know this material.

  There will be questions on the examination that I can't answer.

  I will let my study group down.

- Develop your plan by:

  Setting realistic goals for yourself.

  Defining how much time each goal will take to realize.

  Building in rewards.

  Building in time for review.

  Fantasizing – see yourself succeeding!

- Admit to mistakes:

  Everyone makes them, it is part of the learning experience.

  Distractions - build extra time into your study schedule, and try to re-focus on the task.

  Emotion – we all get frustrated at times, especially when things are not going as well as we had planned. Turn that frustration around, and acknowledge that you are doing something about it.

Index Study Systems

Using index study systems is an effective strategy to evaluate how well you know and understand the material you have studied. Follow these steps to build up your own index study system:

- As you read through your study notes, write down potential test questions about the material on one side of an index card:

  What activities are likely to be affected for a data entry clerk who has de Quervain's Tenosynovitis?

  What kind of splint would be beneficial for an individual with de Quervain's Tenosynovitis?

  How should the worksite be modified to assist this individual?

- On the other side of the card, write an explanation to answer your questions. Include references or texts you have used during your studying to validate your response.

  Individuals with de Quervain's Tenosynovitis should avoid thumb flexion and ulnar deviation - encourage neutral positioning split keyboard/modified mouse, handle modifications. A rigid thumb spica splint with thumb immobilized in abduction, wrist in extension.

  (Reference: Burke, Higgins, McClinton, Saunders, Valdata (2006). Hand and Upper Extremity Rehabilitation, a practical guide. (3rd Ed.). St Louis: Elsevier. (pages 441-7).

- When you have completed writing up a series of index cards about a particular subject, shuffle the cards. Look at the card on top and read the question. Try to answer it in your own words. If you experience difficulty, turn the card over and review the answer you have written.

- Keep going through the deck until you know all the information you have catalogued.

- Carry the cards with you – take advantage of free time to review your knowledge.

- Use the cards to study with your peer group. Test each other, check that others understand your explanations, come up with alternative solutions to the problems posted.

Cooperative and Collaborative Learning

Your occupational therapy education has provided many opportunities for you to experience cooperative and collaborative learning opportunities. This is an interactive learning approach where group members develop and share a common goal, contribute understanding of specific problems, post questions, offer insights and solutions. Many students find it effective to use a similar approach for studying to take the certification examination.

What makes an effective study group?
- Use understanding of group process principles.
- Keep the group to a manageable size (maximum of six).
- Assign a group leader.
- Choose members who will bring specific strengths to the group.
- Empower members to contribute.
- Encourage commitment.
- Share group operating principles and responsibilities such as:
  - Commitment to attend, preparation, and starting meetings on time.
  - Having discussions and disagreements that focus on issues, not personal criticism.
  - Taking responsibility to share tasks and carry them out on time.

Process of setting up a study group:
- Set goals, define how often and with what means you will communicate, evaluate progress, make decisions, and resolve conflict.
- Define resources, especially someone who can provide direction, supervision, counsel, and even arbitrate.
- Schedule review of your progress and communication to discuss what is working, and what is not working.

Test-Taking Strategies

*S*ection II presented an array of strategies to encourage effective study habits. This next section examines general test-taking strategies including what to do before, during, and after the test, tips for overcoming test anxiety, and guidelines for answering multiple-choice items.

Before, During, and After the Test

Before the test:

Remind yourself of the progress you have made to date. You have already completed an occupational therapy program. You have taken many academic courses, successfully completed assignments, and passed several major tests. Think back to how much you knew about occupational therapy at the start of your program, compared to how much you know now. View the certification examination as just one step further towards your goal of becoming an occupational therapy practitioner. You have taken many steps up to this point, and this is one of the last steps you will need to take towards your career goal.

Continue to set realistic study goals, identifying your strengths and addressing any weaknesses in your knowledge. Use the Examination Readiness Tool in Appendix A to help you. Regularly review your progress, check off your study goals, seek additional help for information you are finding difficult to understand, build in regular breaks, and try to predict how the information you are studying might be presented on the test. Remember that items on the certification examination are always practice-based. Regularly demonstrate the knowledge you have acquired through: revising your study notes, using index systems, contributing to a study group, using lists, charts, and writing review papers.

The night before the test:

- Do not engage in last minute cramming. If you have followed a well-planned study schedule, there is no need for you to do last minute cramming.
- Make sure you know the exact site of the examination center. Estimate how long it will take you to get there and build in extra time for traffic, taking the wrong turn, unforeseen circumstances. Make sure your vehicle has gas, and is in full working order.
- Make sure you have all the documentation you will need to take with you to the test site – refer to the latest copy of the NBCOT Candidate Handbook online at www.nbcot.org.
- Pack earplugs to bring along to test site if you feel this will help your concentration as you take the examination.
- Engage in some form of physical activity. This will help to alleviate pretest nerves.
- Decide what clothes you plan to wear – comfort and layered clothing are the key considerations. Try to get a good night's sleep, and remember to set the alarm clock.

The day of the test:

- Arrive at the test site early.
- Try not to talk to others taking the same test – anxiety can be contagious.
- Take some deep, slow breaths.
- Remind yourself how well you have done up to this point.
- Organize your workspace – familiarize yourself with the computer and ensure you can see a watch/ clock.
- Ask for headphones or use your earplugs if you know you will be distracted by others working around you.

- Ensure your seat feels comfortable, and sit in an upright position.
- Advise the test center proctor of any problems or concerns you have regarding the test environment prior to beginning the test.

During the test:
- Divide up your test time carefully. There are 2 sections on the examination – section 1 contains 3 clinical simulation test items and section 2 contains 170 multiple-choice test items.
- Take the tutorials before completing each section of the examination. There is one tutorial before each of the two sections. Time for taking the tutorials is NOT deducted from your actual exam time.
- Use erasable board and marker pen (you can request this at the test site) to help you organize and clarify your thinking.
- Change your position regularly – stretch, drop your shoulders, open and close your fingers, shift in your chair.
- Read the instructions VERY CAREFULLY before answering the test items:
  When answering clinical simulation problems:
  - Remember when you've selected an action you cannot deselect it.
  - You cannot add actions to previous screens once you have progressed to a new screen
  When answering multiple-choice items:
  - Use the "Mark" button on the computer screen to review items later if time permits.
  - Only change an answer you have initially selected if you are really sure it is an incorrect response. The answer that comes to mind first is often correct.
  - Rely on your knowledge and do not watch for patterns. The test answers are randomized.
- Don't panic if other people in the room finish before you do. You do not need to leave the room until you have used all of the allotted time.
- If you experience problems during the exam, inform the test center proctor.

After the test:
- Resist the urge to talk through test items and potential answers with your peer group. You have completed the exam, and it is too late to change your answers now.
- Resist the urge to open up your study notes, texts, and review guides for the same reason given above.
- Remember, it is against NBCOT's Candidate/Certificant Code of Conduct to discuss test items with other candidates, or to record test information from memory.
- Relax. You have waited for this moment for a long time, you can do no more, reward yourself for completing this stage.
- If you do wish to post an exam challenge, ensure you do this in writing, and within the timelines given in the NBCOT Candidate Handbook, and on page 28 of this guide.

Overcoming Test Anxiety

It is of course, very natural to experience a level of anxiety prior to sitting for the certification examination. This is a day that you have been working towards for a long period of time, and marks your passage towards achieving your career goal. Your occupational therapy education has provided you with many instances when anxiety has been a natural response—interviewing your first real patient, arriving at your first day of fieldwork, giving a formal presentation in front of a large audience. Remind yourself that a certain amount of anxiety can actually be very beneficial to your performance. It heightens your awareness and enables you to remain alert. Anxiety can become a problem however, if it lasts too long and starts to interfere with your ability to concentrate.

The following are some tips to help you manage your anxiety:

- Prepare, prepare, prepare. This includes following a realistic and well planned study schedule, as well as preparing physically for getting to the test site on time.
- Ensure you have exercised, eaten, and had a good night's sleep.
- Use cue cards to remind you how well you have done.
- View the test as an opportunity to demonstrate how much you know and have achieved.
- Remember, the examination is not designed to trick you.
- Engage in relaxation techniques – visualization, controlled breathing, tensing and relaxing muscles groups.
- Change position, visit the restroom, have a drink of water.

If you notice that at times you have not been able to manage your anxiety levels, and that this has interfered with your ability to perform on exams, seek help from a qualified professional. Your student counseling center, or healthcare provider will be able to recommend help available to you.

> *Remember, taking the certification examination brings you one step further toward your goal of becoming an occupational therapy practitioner. Remind yourself of the progress you have made to get to this point!*

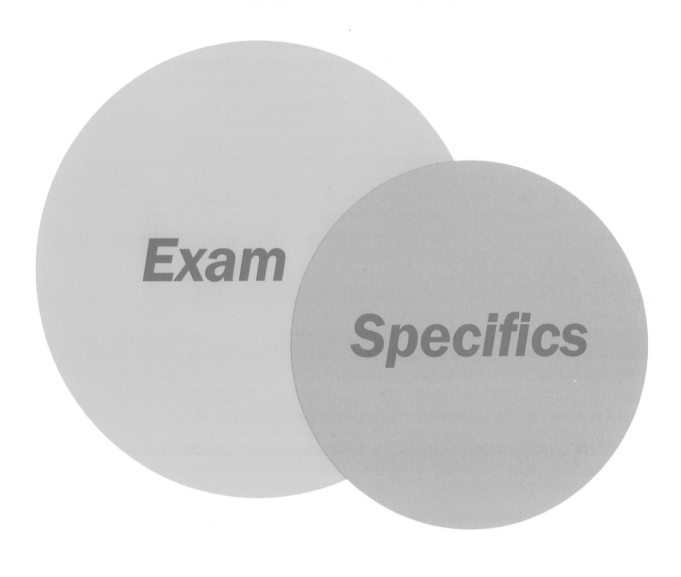

Exam Specifics

Background

Following certification industry standards, NBCOT certification examinations are constructed based on the results of practice analysis studies. The ultimate goal of practice analysis studies are to ensure that there is a representative linkage of test content to practice, making certain that the credentialing examination contains meaningful indicators of competence, and providing evidence that supports the examination's content validity of current occupational therapy practice. The periodic performance of practice analysis studies assists NBCOT with evaluating the validity of the test specifications that guide content distribution of the credentialing examinations. Because the practice of occupational therapy changes and evolves over time, practice analysis studies are conducted by NBCOT on a regular basis.

NBCOT conducted a practice analysis study of OTR practice in 2007. The results from this study were used to construct examination test blueprints for administrations starting January 2009.

Building upon previous studies, a large-scale survey was used with entry-level OTR practitioners who were asked to evaluate job requirements on criticality and frequency rating scales. The job requirements were classified as the domains, tasks, knowledge and skills required for current occupational therapy assistant practice.

- ▣ Domains broadly define the major performance components of the profession.
- ▣ Tasks describe activities that are performed in each domain (i.e., things that practitioners do).
- ▣ Knowledge statements describe the information required to perform each task competently.
- ▣ Skills describe the abilities needed by the Certificant to implement the task. Samples of domain, task, knowledge and skill statements are as follows:

Domain: Gather information regarding factors that influence occupational performance
Task: Identify environments and contexts using appropriate theoretical approaches or models of practice in order to determine facilitators and/or barriers that impact the client's participation in occupation
Knowledge of: Theoretical approaches and models of practice
Skill: Using appropriate theoretical approaches or models of practice to identify environmental and contextual factors that support or hinder occupational performance

The results of the survey were analyzed to identify the most critical and frequently performed tasks by the OTR survey respondents. Weights were then established to determine the relative proportion of test items devoted to each of the four domain areas established for the OTR examination blueprints. Table 4.1 displays the OTR blueprint specifications derived from the results of the 2007 NBCOT practice analysis study. These blueprints will guide examination development for the NBCOT OTR certification examinations beginning January 2009.

The percentage of items in each domain area shown on page 21 remains constant on each exam form of the OTR certification examination. There are multiple task, knowledge, and skill statements for each of the four domain areas. For a full overview of task, knowledge, and skill statements specific to each of the four domain areas for the OTR certification examination, please see Appendix E.

Table 4.1. OTR Blueprint Specifications Based on the 2007 Practice Analysis Study – Implementation January 2009 examination administrations

Domain	Description	Percent of Exam
01	Gather information regarding factors that influence occupational performance	13%
02	Formulate conclusions regarding the client's needs and priorities to develop a client-centered intervention plan	28%
03	Select and implement evidence-based interventions to support participation in areas of occupation (e.g., ADL, education, work, play, leisure, social participation) throughout the continuum of care	39%
04	Uphold professional standards and responsibilities to promote quality in practice	20%

Exam Construction

NBCOT contracts with a professional testing agency who is responsible for meeting test specifications, including item construction, and ensuring that accepted psychometric principles in test construction are met. The testing agency assists NBCOT during test development by assuring the content validity, reliability, and security of the NBCOT examinations.

Each item (question) appearing on the OTR examination has been developed to assess essential knowledge acceptable for entry-level performance by an occupational therapist. In addition, the items are designed to differentiate from an individual whose knowledge is acceptable for certification and an individual whose knowledge is not acceptable for certification. All items have been subjected to multiple rigorous review. Examination items are carefully reviewed for bias, making sure that the context, setting, language, descriptions, terminology, and content of the items are free of stereotype and equally appropriate for all segments of the candidate population.

The OTR examination forms administered from January 2009 onwards will consist of multiple choice and simulation test items (see "Format of the OTR Examination" beginning on page 22 for details). A number of the multiple choice and simulation items are scored and a number of them are unscored. The unscored items are intermingled with the scored items and are indistinguishable to the testing candidate. A scored exam item is an item that is considered in the pass/fail status of a candidate. Each examination item is psychometrically analyzed prior to use on the examination as a scored item. As a matter of practice, examination items are field-tested; however, responses from the field-test items are not included in a candidate's examination score. After field-test items have a fixed number of examination administrations, the items are psychometrically analyzed to determine if they satisfy credentialing standards for valid and reliable test questions. If the items satisfy these standards, they are included in the item bank for future use.

In summary, no scoreable item is included on the certification examination that does not 1) satisfy the examination blueprint specifications resulting from the practice analysis study, 2) meet development standards described above, or 3) satisfy the psychometric standards for a scoreable exam item.

Format of the OTR Examination

From January 2009 onwards the OTR examination will consist of a section of multiple choice test items and a section of clinical simulation test (CST) problems.

Multiple-Choice Test Items

Each multiple-choice test item starts with a stem or premise. This is usually in the form of a written statement or a question. Stems always relate to tasks, knowledge, and skills required for entry-level OTR practice. The following is an example of a stem:

> *A client who is right hand dominant and has mild hemiplegia secondary to a right CVA one week ago will be participating in outpatient OT. The client is a retired professional pianist whose primary goal is to play the piano at a family reunion in 3 months time. Which activity is **BEST** to include as part of the client's intervention?*

Following the stem, there are four possible response options. From the four options, there is only ONE correct response, the other three options are distractors. It may be that all the responses provided are plausible to some degree, but there is only one choice that is the **BEST** response. Candidates need to solicit the best response based on all the information presented in the stem. The following are the four possible response options posted for the example above:

> A. *Turning pages in a music book to select music pieces for a former colleague to perform at the event*
> B. *Bearing weight through the right arm on the piano stool while using the left hand to play a tune on the piano*
> C. *Integrating piano keyboard drills into a repetitive upper extremity exercise program*
> D. *Listening to favorite piano music while completing dominance retraining activities*

In considering the response options provided, the candidate should ask, "What is this question *really* asking?" The question above is testing the candidate's skill to choose an appropriate client-centered activity in order to assist the client to meet the goal of playing the piano at a family reunion. The candidate must also recognize that the client is right hand dominant and has mild heimiplegia in the non-dominant hand. Response option A is incorrect because it does not promote progress toward the client's goal. Although option B is an activity that may help to increase fine motor control of the affected hand during a preferred activity, weight bearing of the non-involved extremity is not indicated. The client is right hand dominant and has left hemiparesis, therefore, dominance retraining is not indicated; making response option D incorrect. Option C is correct because it uses an activity that fits with the client's goal to return to piano-playing.

Although there is never more than one correct answer in a multiple-choice item, candidates may find it difficult to choose between the options. If this is the case re-read the stem and identify the key words such as the "**BEST** response", "**INITIAL** action", "**FIRST** action", or **NEXT** step. This will help you to determine the correct answer.

The following sample item illustrates this:

> *An OTR is interviewing an inpatient who had a total hip replacement 2 days ago. The patient has no interest in talking about home layout and does not want to learn information about adaptive equipment. What **INITIAL** action should the OTR take in this situation?*
>
> A. *Ask the patient open-ended questions to obtain an understanding of the patient's intentions.*
> B. *Explain in more detail the importance of using adaptive equipment during rehabilitation.*
> C. *Reschedule the session at a time when a caregiver is present to learn the information.*
> D. *Respect the patient's wishes and discharge the client from occupational therapy services.*

The correct response is A as this answer supports a collaborative approach during intervention planning and should be the **INITIAL** action that the OTR takes related to the patient's disinterest. Options B and C may be appropriate at a later stage, but they do not address the patient's reasons for not wanting to learn to use adaptive equipment. Option D is incorrect – there is no information contained in the stem to warrant a discharge from occupational therapy services at this stage.

Scenario Formats

Some of the multiple-choice items on the OTR certification examination are grouped together into scenario formats, whereby there is an introductory passage accompanied by several questions that link back to the same passage. The following is an example of a scenario format:

An OTR is evaluating a client who has a 3-month history of insidious onset elbow pain in the dominant extremity. The evaluation results include tenderness on palpation over the origin of the extensor carpi radialis brevis, increased pain on resisted wrist extension, and decreased grip strength on all 5 settings of the dynamometer. The client reports pain is worst after working an 8-hour shift as an assembly line worker.

1. *Which diagnosis is **TYPICALLY** associated with this client's symptoms?*

   A. *Radial tunnel syndrome*
   B. *Carpal tunnel syndrome*
   C. *Lateral epicondylitis**
   D. *DeQuervain's tenosynovitis*

2. *What type of splint/brace would be **MOST BENEFICIAL** for this client?*

   A. *Counter-force brace**
   B. *Thumb-opponens splint*
   C. *Neoprene elbow sleeve*
   D. *Posterior long-arm splint*

3. *Which self-administered intervention would be **MOST EFFECTIVE** for reducing the client's pain at the end of the work shift?*

   A. *Cool water soaks*
   B. *Paraffin baths*
   C. *Heating pad*
   D. *Ice packs**

In answering multiple-choice items in scenario formats, refer back to the introductory passage for key information to assist your decision-making for selecting the correct response. So in the example above, question 2 is testing your knowledge of choosing an appropriate splint/brace for this client. The scenario stem provides key facts about the client's presenting symptoms – tenderness over origin of extensor carpi radialis brevis, pain on resisted wrist extension, and decreased grip strength. Based on this information, the correct response is a counter-force brace as this would be the most beneficial orthoses to use for a client who has symptoms consistent with tennis elbow.

Summary - When answering multiple-choice test items:

- ☐ **Read and re-read the stem or introductory passage.**
- ☐ **Identify the key words.**
- ☐ **Ask yourself, "What is this question really asking?"**
- ☐ **Eliminate the obvious incorrect answers.**
- ☐ **Re-read the information in the stem for clues to determine the correct response.**
- ☐ **Select the best response.**

Clinical Simulation Test Problems

Clinical simulation testing (CST) is a format of assessment designed to replicate the types of situations certified occupational therapy practitioners encounter in their everyday practice. The problems measure a candidate's knowledge and critical reasoning ability sequentially across the continuum of care, for example: screening, formulating treatment needs and priorities; implementing interventions; and assessing outcomes.

Each simulation problem consists of:

a. *An opening scene*
b. *A series of accompanying sections each with section headers*
c. *A list of actions ranging from positive, neutral, or negative responses*

Candidates select the actions that they deem appropriate from the list of actions provided. As the action statement is selected, a feedback box will appear. Feedback is revealed response-by-response as the candidate makes each selection, so that a candidate only receives information on the actions they have chosen throughout the course of the problem.

From the list of actions, a candidate will score points for positive actions and have points deducted for actions that are negative or hinder the resolution of the presented problem(s). A candidate will neither have points awarded nor deducted for selecting a neutral action.

Candidates will have the ability to scroll back through the simulation problem to view:

- ▣ Opening scene
- ▣ Section headers
- ▣ Actions they have selected

This helps candidates to tie decisions to their previous actions. However, once a candidate has progressed to the next screen, they will not be able to add actions to previous screens.

An example of the beginning of a CST problem is shown on page 25.

Summary - When answering simulation test items:

- ▣ A CST problem consists of an opening scene with accompanying linked sections and lists of actions.
- ▣ Refer to key phrases in the opening scene and section headers to help you decide on the appropriate action options to select.
- ▣ Remember, once an action has been selected it cannot be de-selected.
- ▣ As you progress through the CST problem, you can tie your decisions to previous sections by scrolling back to review.
- ▣ You cannot add actions to previous screens once you have progressed to a new screen.

Note the opening scene, section header under section A, list of actions, and feedback accompanying the actions that have been selected.

OPENING SCENE

An OTR working in a school setting receives a referral from a teacher for a seven-year-old student. The teacher is concerned about the student's classroom performance and fine motor skills. A social history reveals that the student has an older sibling who has autism and attends the same school.

Section A

Which actions are appropriate for the OTR to take during the screening process to determine the appropriateness of occupational therapy services for this student? (Choose all of those actions that are appropriate at this time.)

	Action	Outcome
☑	Ask the teacher to identify the student's favorite storybook.	The teacher indicates the student likes The Cat in the Hat stories.
☐	Observe the student participating in classroom activities.	
☐	Complete a review of the student's school health record.	
☐	Confirm the allocation of COTA hours to the school.	
☐	Consult with the school nurse to arrange for an updated visual screening.	
☑	Contact the school district to confirm the number of students currently receiving occupational therapy services at the school.	The school district confirms that 14 students are currently receiving services at the school.
☐	Interview the student's parents.	
☐	Observe the student engaged in a craft activity.	
☐	Determine developmental delays experienced by the student's sibling.	
☐	Review the student's recent written assignments.	
☐	Complete an unstructured observation of the student interacting with family members in the home environment.	
	Next	

It is IMPORTANT to note, once an action has been selected on the computer, that particular action cannot be de-selected.

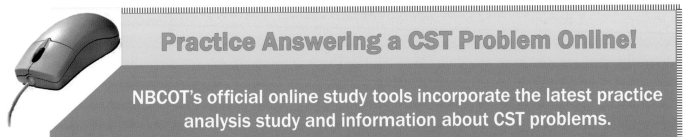

Practice Answering a CST Problem Online!

NBCOT's official online study tools incorporate the latest practice analysis study and information about CST problems.

To learn more about CST formats and to purchase a practice test containing CST problems, please visit *www.nbcot.org*.

Standard Setting, Equating, & Scoring

All NBCOT certification examinations are criterion referenced. This means in order to pass the examination, the candidate must obtain a score equal to – or higher than – the minimum passing score. The minimum passing score represents an absolute standard and does not depend on the performance of other candidates taking the same examination. The minimum passing score on the OTR certification examination is set by content experts using widely recognized standard setting methodologies.

NBCOT develops multiple forms of their certification examinations to ensure security and integrity of the examination. Every form employs a unique combination of test items so that no two forms are identical but all forms are equal in difficulty level.

NBCOT uses a scaled scoring procedure to determine a candidate's final score. The scaled score is not a "number correct" or "percent correct" score. Raw scores are converted to scale scores that represent equivalent levels of achievement regardless of test form. The passing point for NBCOT's OTR certification examination is set at 450 points with the lowest possible score set at 300 and the highest possible score set at 600 points. Candidates must obtain a scaled score of at least 450 points in order to pass the examination. For more information on the psychometric principles that form the foundations of the NBCOT certification examinations, please refer to *www.nbcot.org*.

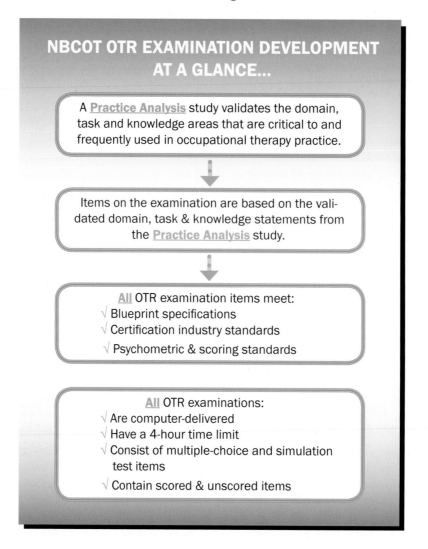

NBCOT OTR EXAMINATION DEVELOPMENT AT A GLANCE...

A **Practice Analysis** study validates the domain, task and knowledge areas that are critical to and frequently used in occupational therapy practice.

Items on the examination are based on the validated domain, task & knowledge statements from the **Practice Analysis** study.

All OTR examination items meet:
√ Blueprint specifications
√ Certification industry standards
√ Psychometric & scoring standards

All OTR examinations:
√ Are computer-delivered
√ Have a 4-hour time limit
√ Consist of multiple-choice and simulation test items
√ Contain scored & unscored items

Examination Preparation Tools

In addition to this study guide, NBCOT has developed a number of resources to assist examination candidates with their test preparation, for example the OTR Exam Readiness Tool (see Appendix A) and online OTR practice tests. All official NBCOT study tools are developed to meet the current examination blueprint specifications with items that have been developed in the same manner as those used on the actual certification examination. For details of the official NBCOT study tools, visit *www.nbcot.org*.

TEST ADMINISTRATION

Taking Computer-Based Tests

Test centers are built to standard specifications and vary primarily on the basis of size. NBCOT candidates arriving at the test site must have a valid, current, government-issued ID, and must sign the roster. Private modular workstations provide ample workspace, comfortable seating, and lighting. Proctors monitor the testing process through an observation window and from within the testing room. Parabolic mirrors mounted on the walls assist proctors in observing the testing process. All testing sessions are videotaped and audio-monitored. During the testing session, people taking examinations other than the NBCOT examinations may be in the testing room.

The test is administered at a standard work station. The regular computer table/desks are about 28" (71 cm) from the floor. All of the chairs are adjustable in height from at least 15 1/2" from the floor to 20 1/2" (39-52 cm). Some chairs have even more range than that. Chairs do have armrests. Every site has 2-foot (61 cm) stools available to candidates should feet not reach the floor with chair adjustment. The monitors can be pointed upward or downward, or turned from one side to another. Should the initial monitor placement result in glare, an adjustment such as this will resolve that issue.

The examination consists of two sections: section one contains 3 clinical simulation problems and section two contains 170 multiple-choice test items. There is a tutorial before EACH section of the examination explaining the process of selecting responses to the examination items. Time spent on the tutorials does NOT count against the time allotted for the examination. Candidates are strongly encouraged to take the tutorials prior to starting each section of the examination. Candidates are allotted four (4) hours to complete the examination.

A standard 14-point font is used for the screen text. When answering clinical simulation test items, use the scroll bar on the right of the screen to review all the options listed in the decision/action lists. Once an action has been selected, it cannot be deselected. Once you have progressed to the next screen, you are not able to add actions to previous screens. During the multiple-choice section of the examination, you can use the "Mark" and "Unmark" buttons to flag items, and the "Review" button to return to marked items if time permits. If you run out of time, marked items that have responses will be counted for scoring purposes.

All test situations are subject to some noise and distraction. In a computer-based setting, other test-takers may be taking essay exams, so there may be some keyboarding sounds from test-takers nearby. The test center staff may also be providing some brief assistance to other test-takers in the room. If a candidate is concerned that these situations may be distracting, earplugs are permitted. Candidates are allowed to use earplugs that are supplied by the testing center, or they may bring their own. Earplugs are not automatically distributed to candidates. Candidates must ask test center staff for them. However, because there is no guarantee of the availability of earplugs, candidates who believe that they will need earplugs are strongly advised to bring their own. Note that only small "in-the-ear" earplugs are allowed. Large "room silencers" or any headphone-types of equipment are not allowed without prior special accommodations approval.

Candidates may stop and take a break, go to the restroom, or get some water or a snack from a locker. Breaks may be taken at any time, and as often as is reasonable and necessary. The exam time continues to run during any breaks. For more details on test administration, refer to the current copy of the NBCOT Certification Examination Handbook.

Accommodations

In compliance with the Americans with Disabilities Act (ADA), NBCOT makes special testing arrangements for candidates with professionally diagnosed and documented disabilities. Under the ADA, a disability is defined as "a physical or mental impairment that substantially limits one or more major life activities" (e.g., caring for one's self, performing manual tasks, walking, seeing, breathing, learning, working). If you intend to apply for special testing accommodations in order to take the COTA certification examination, you need to provide comprehensive documentation supporting your diagnosis, and the impact of the disability on major life activity. Submit the documentation AFTER you have filed your examination application. A review is then conducted per ADA guidelines. An Authorization to Test (ATT) letter will be sent only after the decision about the special accommodations request is final. Please refer to information about Special Accommodations online at *www.nbcot.org*.

Unfortunate Events

Examination Content Challenges, Administration Complaints, and Appeals
A candidate may challenge the content of specific test items (include as much specific information as possible about the test item) or file a complaint regarding the administration of the examination by sending a letter describing the basis for the content challenge or administrative complaint and including pertinent information. The letter of challenge or complaint must be POSTMARKED NO LATER THAN 24 HOURS AFTER THE CANDIDATE TAKES THE EXAMINATION AND SENT VIA TRACEABLE MAIL/DELIVERY – SIGNATURE OF RECEIPT REQUIRED (e.g., certified mail) to NBCOT.

With regard to a letter of administrative complaint or content challenge, NBCOT will investigate and respond in writing to the candidate. A candidate may appeal the decision by sending a letter describing the justification of the appeal. This letter of appeal must be received by NBCOT no later than 21 days after the candidate's receipt of the notification of NBCOT's decision. Please refer to the latest NBCOT Candidate Handbook online at *www.nbcot.org*.

Failing the Examination

Unfortunately, not every candidate who takes NBCOT's certification examinations will achieve a successful passing score. While it is obviously very disappointing to receive notification that you did not meet the passing requirement (a scaled score of 450 points or above), it is essential to address the consequences of this occurrence. A candidate's test score (including a fail score) will only be reported to the candidate, and to a state licensing board, if the candidate requested for their score transfer reports to be sent to a state regulatory board(s). **Without the candidate's written permission, no other persons will be informed of the candidate's failed score.** Not passing the NBCOT certification examination may impact the candidate's plans to commence an occupational therapy job position. It is the candidate's responsibility to inform any potential employer that they are not currently certified, if they did not successfully pass the NBCOT certification examination and are seeking employment as an OTR. Candidates need to contact state regulatory entities for specific information regarding temporary licenses.

Candidates who fail the certification examination will be informed as to when they are able to schedule a subsequent examination within a specific examination eligibility period. The eligibility period can begin no sooner than 45 days from the test date shown on the candidate's score report. A new Authorization to Test (ATT) letter will be sent to the candidate and this will specify the next examination eligibility period based on the 45-day end-date and receipt of the new application.

Preparing to Re-Take the Certification Examination

There may be many reasons for a candidate failing NBCOT's certification examination. Reflecting on potential reasons is an important first step in preparing to re-take the examination. These reasons may include:

- Poor test-taking strategies
- Inadequate study habits
- Lack of preparation
- Test anxiety
- External stresses

After identifying potential reasons, revisit the initial sections in this study guide to help develop a plan of action. Pay particular attention to the sections on Adult Learning, Developing Effective Study Habits, and General Test-Taking Strategies. Use the sample multiple-choice items at the end of this study guide to help familiarize yourself with the format and domain areas of the certification examination. For any incorrect responses, use the rationales and follow-up references to help guide your study and preparation.

Interpreting The Score Reports

Candidates who fail the NBCOT OTR certification examination will be provided with a score report that outlines the candidate's scaled score for each of the domain areas represented in the certification examination. In addition, information regarding the average U.S. new graduate candidate's scaled scores across domains is also included.

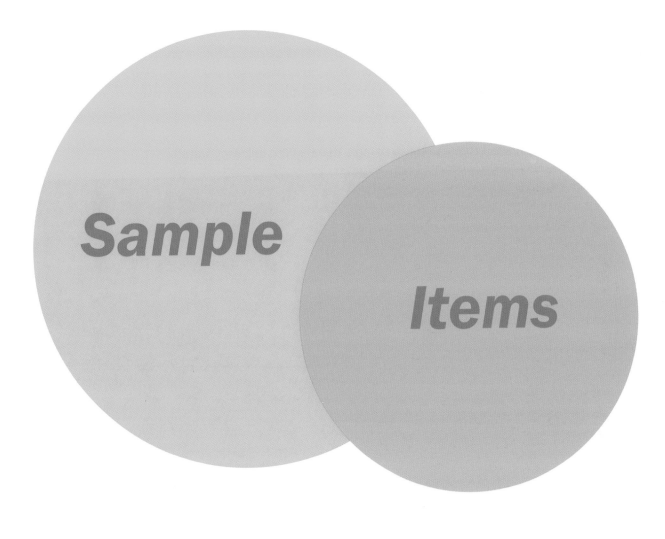

Multiple-Choice Sample Items

The 2007 Blueprint Specifications for the OTR validated domain, task, and knowledge statements (see Appendix E) provides the basis for the OTR certification examination item development. The outline for the examination is based upon the four domain areas identified in the blueprint, and the percentage for each domain weight (the approximate percent of items from the domain appearing on each examination) is listed on page 21.

This section consists of 100 OTR multiple-choice sample items across all four domain areas. Examples of domain-specific test items are grouped together under each domain heading for learning purposes in this study guide. However, candidates should take note that the items on the actual certification examination will appear in random order.

It is recommended that candidates use these sample items in the following ways:

- Start by completing the Examination Readiness Tool in Appendix A. This will highlight areas of strength and weakness.
- Next, read and answer the sample items. As a guide to develop an effective study plan, identify items that you score incorrectly. Read the rationale for the correct response, and follow up by studying the reference materials listed.
- Practice taking a timed test. The actual certification exam will contain one section of 170 multiple choice items (multiple choice and scenario items) plus 3 clinical simulation problems. Unless you have been granted special accommodations, you will be allotted a total of four hours for the entire examination. Take this into consideration as you divide your time up for the practice test.
- Use the 2007 Blueprint Specifications (Appendix E) to identify specific domain areas with subsequent task and knowledge statements to enhance your studying and preparation efforts.
- After answering the sample items, compare your answers to the answer key on page 58.
- For incorrect answers, refer to the answer section beginning on page 59. Read the rationale for the correct answer and explanations for the incorrect answers. Use the references provided for additional information to enhance your studying.
- Use this experience to guide discussion in your study groups or further guide individual examination preparation efforts.

The following multiple-choice items are samples related to Domain Area 1:

Gather information regarding factors that influence occupational performance

1. A second-grade student is being evaluated by an OT due to difficulty completing assigned art and writing activities. Standardized assessment results indicate the student has age-appropriate comprehension, visual object gnosia, and visual acuity, but scores on figure-ground subtests are well below the norm. Problems associated with this perceptual skill would be **MOST EVIDENT** during which of the following art activities?

    A. Free-form painting of a clay pot with a variety of paint colors
    B. Selecting a round bead from a bag of multi-shaped beads to complete a necklace
    C. Using plastic templates to trace basic geometric shapes on colored paper
    D. Placing tiles of the same color and shape in a straight line when making a trivet

2. Which dressing task requires the **MOST** challenging integration of performance skills and patterns for a typically developing 3-year-old child?

    A. Finding armholes in a pull-over shirt – 2
    B. Unfastening the zipper of a front-opening jacket – 3 – 3½
    C. Pulling down a pair of elastic waist pants – 2½
    D. Pulling off a pair of ankle-high socks – (younger old)

3. An OTR is completing an initial evaluation of a 4-year-old child who has moderate cerebral palsy. A neuro-motor assessment indicates that primitive reflexes dominate the child's movement patterns, and abnormal oral motor control interferes with feeding and functional communication. What additional information is **MOST IMPORTANT** for the OTR to collect prior to developing an intervention plan?

    A. Contextual features that support the child's typical participation in occupation
    B. Evaluation reports from other professionals involved with the child's rehabilitation
    C. Early intervention programs available for supporting the child's academic readiness
    D. Medical reports that include the child's past medical history and developmental prognosis

4. An OTR is a contributing investigator in a unit-wide research project. The focus of the project is to determine if participation in rehabilitation is beneficial to a client's health, well-being, and general quality of life. Which of the following standardized assessment tools would be **MOST EFFECTIVE** for the OTR to use for this study?

    A. Short Form-36 Health Survey (SF-36)
    B. Kohlman Evaluation of Living Skills (KELS)
    C. Functional Independence Measure (FIM)
    D. Barthel Index of ADL

Sample Items

5.   An OTR is preparing to evaluate a young adult client who recently sustained traumatic bilateral above knee amputations. The OTR wants to identify the client's priorities and personal goals regarding engagement in daily activities. Which of the following assessment tools would be **MOST BENEFICIAL** for the OTR to use?

A.   Kohlman Evaluation of Living Skills (KELS)
B.   Functional Independence Measure (FIM)
C.   Role Checklist
D.   Canadian Occupational Performance Measure (COPM)

6.   A client who has had a mild acquired brain injury is participating in a work readiness program. The client's goal is to resume work as a professional chef in a restaurant where he worked prior to the accident. Which context is **BEST** for observing the client's skills and abilities?

A.   In the client's home kitchen with familiar surroundings
B.   In the kitchen of a culinary arts technical training school
C.   In the kitchen of the restaurant where the client will work
D.   In the OT kitchen in the rehabilitation center

7.   A client who has had a CVA is preparing for discharge from an inpatient rehabilitation facility to home. The client is independent with BADL, and the OTR has completed a visit to the client's home. Which of the following constructs represents the ecology of human performance approach and should be reflected in the client's discharge summary?

A.   Recommendations for home modifications to maximize accessibility and task performance
B.   Exercise protocols for maintaining physical strength and cardiovascular endurance
C.   Current functional status and anticipated occupational performance upon return home
D.   Recommended community support groups and resources to promote adaptation to physical impairments

8.   An OTR is developing an intervention plan using a bottom-up approach for clients who have chronic hemiplegia and hemi-neglect. Which of the following intervention techniques uses this approach and has evidence supporting its efficacy for reducing the effects of "learned non-use" through cortical reorganization?

A.   Proprioceptive neuromuscular facilitation
B.   Neurodevelopmental training
C.   Occupational adaptation
D.   Constraint-induced therapy

9. An OTR is preparing to complete an initial grooming and hygiene assessment of an inpatient who has had a CVA, and has recently been transferred to an inpatient rehabilitation facility. Where is the **BEST** location for the OTR to complete the assessment?

   A. At the patient's bedside
   B. In an area of the patient's choosing
   C. In the bathroom of the patient's room
   D. In a simulated environment in the OT clinic

10. A client who sustained a humeral shaft fracture 6 weeks ago was referred to OT with a consult that states: "Begin AROM of the elbow and shoulder". The OTR observes that in addition to elbow and shoulder stiffness, the client's hand is minimally swollen and has full passive ROM, but the client is unable to actively extend the wrist or digits. What action should the OTR take **INITIALLY** based on these findings?

    A. Include aggressive strengthening of the hand and wrist in the intervention plan.
    B. Determine if the client sustained a radial nerve palsy secondary to the fracture.
    C. Fabricate a dynamic splint to compensate for loss of finger extension.
    D. Complete a manual muscle test to determine the overall strength of the arm.

11. During an initial screening, a client who is in the early stages of multiple sclerosis reports that engaging in daily routines causes exhaustion. The client's goal is to remain independent with homemaking tasks for a family of four, which includes a spouse and two adolescent children. Which of the following should the OTR do **FIRST** as part of the initial evaluation?

    A. Obtain a standardized measure the client's functional independence.
    B. Administer standardized assessments of client factors.
    C. Collaborate with the family regarding typical occupational roles.
    D. Complete a client-centered occupational profile.

12. An OTR is using an adaptive approach with a client who has had a recent acquired brain injury. The client currently has full functional ROM and strength, but a residual visual and vestibular processing deficit interferes with performance in areas of occupation. Which activity incorporates this approach and could be used as part of the client's intervention?

    A. Providing the client with an exercise program for improving gaze stabilization
    B. Teaching the client to use proprioceptive cues during functional activities
    C. Incorporating progressively more challenging tasks into a functional activity
    D. Engaging the client in valued activities that promote postural stability and balance

13. An inpatient who had a total hip replacement several days ago is being taught how to use assistive devices. Neither the patient nor the spouse appear interested in learning how to use the devices. What action should the OTR take based on this observation?

    A. Explore the couple's feelings about using the equipment.
    B. Explain that assistive devices are essential to the patient's recovery.
    C. Advise the patient that the equipment will hasten the healing time.
    D. Document the reactions client's record and inform the care coordinator.

14. An OTR who uses an ecological intervention model is developing an activity program for elderly clients who will be participating in a partial-hospitalization program. Which of the following methods **BEST** represents this approach to intervention program planning?

    A. Selecting activity protocols to promote the clients' participation in a group activity
    B. Interviewing families and caregivers about their expectations and preferences
    C. Coordinating with other professionals about activity choices and client scheduling
    D. Identifying contexts that support the clients' engagement in valued tasks

15. During which kitchen task would deficits related to constructional apraxia be **MOST** evident?

    A. Peeling vegetables
    B. Preparing a sandwich
    C. Stirring cake batter
    D. Pouring milk into a glass

16. An OTR is preparing to evaluate an inpatient who has a TBI and is functioning at Level III on the Rancho Los Amigos scale. Which of the following should the OTR include as part of the **INITIAL** assessment?

    A. Self-care potential screening
    B. Upper extremity manual muscle testing
    C. Standardized visual-perceptual test
    D. Measured responsiveness to objective stimuli

17. What is a critical functional difference **TYPICALLY** observed in a client who has a complete C_6 spinal cord injury compared to a client who has a complete C_5 spinal cord injury?

    A. Improved gross grasp from innervation of the extrinsic flexors
    B. Ability to use triceps strength during transfers
    C. Improved trunk control to bend side to side without falling
    D. Ability to use the radial wrist extensors to supplement grasp

18. Which of the following evaluation methods is **MOST RELIABLE** to use for monitoring hand edema in a client who has hemiplegia?

   A. Circumferential taping
   B. Hand outlines
   C. Volumetric measurements
   D. Clinical observations

19. A patient is in a skilled nursing facility after having had a recent CVA. The client has moderate hemiplegia, uses a quad cane during ambulation, and has good memory. Nursing staff reports that the patient has difficulty finding the way from the dayroom to the dining room despite being shown several times. What should the OTR include in the evaluation based on this report?

   A. A functional assessment of topographical orientation and visual perception
   B. A standardized test containing an attention and a depth perception subtest
   C. A dressing task to assess ideomotor and constructional praxis
   D. An assessment of executive function using an ADL task

20. An OTR wants to complete a standardized visual perceptual evaluation with a client who has had a right CVA. A deficit in which of the following areas would have the **MOST** impact on attaining accurate results when conducting this evaluation?

   A. Pre-morbid visual foundation skills
   B. Long term memory skills
   C. Right-left scanning abilities
   D. Problem solving abilities

21. An OTR is evaluating a client who has an ulnar nerve injury at the wrist level of the right dominant extremity. During which task would this injury be **MOST** evident?

   A. Carrying a briefcase
   B. Turning a key in the car ignition
   C. Operating a desktop calculator
   D. Holding coins in the palm of the hand

22. Which of the following represents an occupation-based top-down approach to intervention for a client who has unilateral neglect?

   A. Teaching a client scanning techniques and adapting the client's home environment
   B. Having the client repetitively practice head turning to find an object placed near the affected side
   C. Placing commonly used toiletry items to the client's affected side for use during a self-care task
   D. Providing tactile-kinesthetic guiding to a client's involved extremity during a dressing task

The following multiple-choice items are samples related to Domain Area 2:

Formulate conclusions regarding the client's needs and priorities to develop a client-centered intervention plan

23. An OTR is developing a program for clients who are scheduled to have bariatric surgery. Which of the following topics represents the effective use of an occupational science perspective for this program?

    A. Self-actualization
    B. Stress management
    C. Lifestyle redesign
    D. Coping with change

24. An inpatient who has had bilateral above-knee (AK) amputations is preparing for discharge to live at home with the spouse and an adult son. The patient has good balance and Fair plus (3+/5) upper extremity strength, is independent with bed mobility and self-care using adaptive equipment, and requires stand-by assistance during transfers and with wheelchair management. The patient's bathroom and home entrance has been modified. What type of information is **MOST IMPORTANT** for the caregivers to learn prior to the patient's return home?

    A. Methods for improving the patient's independence with transfers
    B. Techniques the patient uses to transfer to a variety of surfaces
    C. Energy conservation techniques for the patient to use during ADL
    D. Wrapping techniques for shaping and protecting the residual limb

25. An OTR has completed an evaluation on a young adult who has substance abuse disorder. Results indicate the client has maintained sobriety and steady employment for the past six months, but continues to have an unrealistic self-concept, decreased socialization, and inadequate independent living skills. Which of the following objectives should be included as part of the client's **INITIAL** intervention plan for supporting participation in occupations?

    A. Transition to independent living with a supportive friend
    B. Acquisition of practical skills for basic life management
    C. Engagement in leisure activities with social acquaintances
    D. Education about work stressor that contribute to relapse

26. An individual who has rheumatoid arthritis is referred to an arthritis self-help class. After interviewing and observing the individual, the OTR determines that bilateral hand splints would be beneficial. Which of the following actions should the OTR take **FIRST** based on this finding?

    A. Obtain authorization from the insurance company to fabricate the splints.
    B. Schedule an appointment with the individual to fabricate the splints.
    C. Contact the referring individual's physician to request a consult.
    D. Advise the individual to obtain a consult for splinting from the family physician.

27. An OTR has completed an evaluation of a client who has amyotrophic lateral sclerosis. When reviewing the results of upper extremity goniometric measurements, the OTR notes that the client's active ROM is significantly less than passive ROM. What should the OTR conclude is the **PRIMARY** cause for this discrepancy?

   A. Fasiculations
   B. Bony ankylosis
   C. Soft-tissue shortening
   D. Muscular weakness

28. A client is in the recovery phase of intervention after having had an acute onset of Guillain Barré syndrome one month ago. The OTR advises the client that using assistive devices will improve independence, but the client refuses to use the devices stating: "My wife is happy to help me whenever I need it." How should the OTR respond to the client's comment?

   A. Convince the client to try at least one device.
   B. Discuss the comment with family members.
   C. Respect the client's rights and discharge the client.
   D. Use other techniques to maximize independence.

29. A young adult sustained a crush injury to the forearm two weeks ago resulting in an axonotmesis of the ulnar nerve. The client was referred to OT with a consult that reads: "Evaluate and treat". After obtaining baseline assessment information, which technique is **MOST IMPORTANT** to teach to the client during the initial phase of rehabilitation?

   A. Visual compensation
   B. Hand-dominance retraining
   C. Isometric strengthening
   D. Sensory re-education

30. An OTR is assessing the reflexes of a 4-month-old infant. The OTR places the infant in sitting and encourages the infant to actively flex the neck forward to look at an object held near the infant's chest. Which of the following responses indicates the presence of the symmetrical tonic neck reflex?

   A. Flexion of the upper extremities and extension of the lower extremities
   B. Flexion in both the upper and lower extremities
   C. Flexion of the lower extremities and extension of the upper extremities
   D. Extension of both the upper and lower extremities

31. An OTR is developing intervention goals for a patient who has a TBI, is functioning at Level II on the Rancho Los Amigos scale, and is in the medical treatment phase of recovery. Which statement reflects an appropriate goal for the patient to achieve in three weeks?

   A. "The patient will respond to cueing during personal hygiene tasks without displaying verbal outbursts."
   B. "The patient will use compensatory cognitive strategies to arrive to therapy sessions on-time."
   C. "The patient will follow graphic illustrations to complete dressing tasks within one hour each morning."
   D. "The patient will respond in less than 15 seconds to graded sensory stimulation at least 75% of the time."

32. A client who has a C_7 spinal cord injury has been admitted to an inpatient rehabilitation facility and is beginning OT. One of the client's goals is to be able to prepare family meals. What **INITIAL** action should the OTR take to maximize progress toward this goal?

   A. Observe the client during a standardized meal preparation task.
   B. Assess current physical skills and abilities during a kitchen task.
   C. Identify the client's typical mealtime routines and habits.
   D. Provide the client with assistive devices to use in the kitchen.

33. An inpatient who has flaccid hemiplegia and dysphagia is participating in an interdisciplinary rehabilitation program. One of the intervention goals for this patient is to maximize independence for self-feeding and safety when eating. What information about the patient is **MOST IMPORTANT** for the OTR to present to the team during each care coordination meeting?

   A. Improvements in upper extremity movement patterns used for self-feeding feeding
   B. Specific evidence-based techniques that are being used during intervention sessions
   C. Positioning, adaptive devices and caregiver assistance needed during mealtimes
   D. Ability to select nutritious foods from the hospital dining menu that are safe to swallow

34. An OTR is developing an intervention plan for a client who is in the acute manic phase of bipolar disorder. Which of the following strategies should be included as part of the **INITIAL** intervention plan?

   A. Structuring the environment to encourage creativity and self-expression
   B. Minimizing distractions in the environment to support occupational performance
   C. Arranging a group discussion about the consequences of mania on participation in occupations
   D. Providing opportunities for the client to lead an occupation-based goal-setting group

35. A student who has mild autism and is in the second grade is scheduled to begin school-based OT. The student has difficulty attending to academic tasks and displays tactile defensiveness when in close proximity to other people. Which intervention environment would be **MOST EFFECTIVE** for the majority of this student's intervention sessions?

    A. In a self-contained occupational therapy treatment room
    B. On the playground in an area separated from peers
    C. In the gymnasium when other students are not present
    D. In the classroom during routine classroom activities

36. An outpatient who has an acquired brain injury has been making slow and steady progress toward long-term goals. Over the past several weeks, there has been a decline in the patient's energy level, ability to concentrate, and interest in intervention activities. When asked about the change, the patient replies: "I just can't sleep at night, thinking about the burden I am to my family." What **INITIAL** action should the OTR take based on the patient's current status?

    A. Consult with the patient's primary physician
    B. Advise the patient to consult with a psychiatrist
    C. Adjust the timeframes for achieving short-term goals
    D. Focus on functional progress to motivate the patient

37. An OTR is interpreting scores of a developmental test that was administered to a 3-year-old child. The child scored at the 89th percentile for the child's age and gender group. What can the OTR conclude based on this score?

    A. The child has minor developmental deficits compared to the standardization sample group.
    B. Eleven per cent of the children in the standardization sample scored higher than this child.
    C. This child displays above-average developmental skills compared to a variety of similar children.
    D. These scores are sensitive for measuring small changes in the child's overall development.

38. A young adult who was recently discharged from an inpatient facility following a first episode of a major depression is referred to a community based OT program. The evaluation results indicate the client has decreased concentration, poor personal hygiene, and limited self-assessment skills. One of the client's goals is to learn a job skill. Which opportunity should the OTR provide to the client to promote **INITIAL** progress toward this goal?

    A. Temporary work in a sheltered environment
    B. Transitional employment placement
    C. Exploration of work habits and current abilities
    D. Traditional pre-employment experiences

39. An OTR is completing a meal preparation assessment with a client who has a frontal lobe TBI. The client has good bilateral motor control, but has residual problems with executive functioning. After preparing the meal, the client recognizes that the kitchen area needs to be cleaned, but does not know how to go about doing this. Which mental functions client factor appears **MOST** affected based on this behavior?

    A. Emergent awareness
    B. Selective attention
    C. Episodic memory
    D. Environmental gnosia

40. Which of the following information is **MOST IMPORTANT** to include in a home program for individuals who have acute complex regional pain syndrome (CRPS) of the hand?

    A. Illustrations for performing passive ROM for each joint on the affected hand
    B. Recommendations for minimizing the use of the affected hand during ADL
    C. Instructions for controlling edema and maintaining active ROM
    D. Examples for incorporating energy conservation into daily tasks

41. An OTR is evaluating a client who has a peripheral neuropathy. The OTR notes thenar muscle atrophy, inability to pick up small objects - such as a key or coin from a table top - and decreased grip and tip pinch strength. On which part of the client's hand should the OTR expect to find sensory disturbances when completing a sensory evaluation?

    A. Dorsum of the hand and the dorsal surface of the thumb
    B. Volar surface of the thumb, index, long, and radial half of the ring fingers
    C. Entire palm and tips of the index, long, ring, and small fingers
    D. Volar and dorsal surfaces of the small finger and radial half of the ring finger

42. A client who has a C_6 ASIA A complete tetrapelgia is scheduled to participate in OT. The client's short-term goal is to be able to independently complete as many BADL tasks as possible. Which approach would be effective to use as the **PRIMARY** intervention strategy for promoting initial progress toward the client's goals?

    A. Behavioral
    B. Remedial
    C. Biomechanical
    D. Compensatory

43. A client who is recovering from a severe hand injury reports that family responsibilities makes it impossible to complete the prescribed exercise program and splinting regimen. What **INITIAL** action should the OTR take based on this report?

    A. Determine a home program that fits the client's daily routine.
    B. Analyze a 24-hour log to determine time management issues.
    C. Advise the client to make the home program the highest priority.
    D. Suggest a compensatory approach for dealing with residual deficits.

44. An elder client who has been on prolonged bed rest due to general medical-surgical post-operative complications now has moderate-severe debilitation. The client has been referred to OT to increase strength and endurance for BADL. Initial evaluation results indicate that the client has full passive ROM and Fair minus (3-/5) functional muscle strength of the upper extremities. Which of the following activities would be **MOST DIFFICULT** for this client to complete while seated in a wheelchair?

    A. Crossing one leg over the other to put on loose-fitting slip-on shoes
    B. Putting on a front opening shirt after reaching for the shirt off a bedside stand
    C. Getting a pair of pants that are hanging in the closet and putting them on
    D. Washing hands at a sink and drying the hands using a towel placed next to the sink

45. An adolescent who has a conduct disorder has recently been admitted to an inpatient psychiatric unit. Evaluation results indicate that the adolescent has a poor self-concept, decreased fine and gross motor coordination, and is socially aggressive. What should be the **INITIAL** focus of intervention for this adolescent?

    A. Presenting options for pre-vocational exploration and practice
    B. Encouraging participation in self-expression group activities
    C. Providing opportunities for success in a consistent structured environment
    D. Enhancing physical abilities for completing responsibilities at home

46. An OTR is completing a feeding evaluation of a 4-year-old child who has mild hypotonia, immature oral motor control, and oral hypersensitivity. The child sits in a standard dining chair during meals and requires moderate to maximum assistance from a caregiver for feeding. When attempting to swallow food the child hyperextends the neck, elevates both shoulders, and has poor lip closure. What should the OTR **INITIALLY** teach to the caregiver based on this observation?

    A. Methods for using cryotherapy to stimulate facial muscles prior to feeding the child
    B. Handling techniques for facilitating full forward neck flexion during feeding
    C. Adaptive positioning techniques for promoting trunk alignment
    D. Neuromuscular facilitation techniques for promoting head and trunk stability

SECTION 5

Sample Items

Select and implement evidence-based interventions to support participation in areas of occupation (e.g., ADL, education, work, play, leisure, social participation) throughout the continuum of care

47. An OTR has completed an evaluation of a client who had an open reduction and external fixation of a distal radius fracture several days ago. The client has had swelling, decreased ROM of the digits, and protective posturing of the involved extremity. Which of the following is **MOST IMPORTANT** to include as a part of this client's initial intervention?

    A. Education about proper positioning in a standard pouch sling to minimize swelling
    B. Exercises to promote capsular gliding and ROM of the shoulder of the affected arm
    C. Static splinting to prevent MCP joint collateral ligament tightness
    D. Use of a dry whirlpool modality to manage edema of the affected hand

48. A patient who has flaccid hemiplegia secondary to a CVA is developing edema in the affected hand. Which method should the OTR include as part of the intervention plan for **INITIALLY** managing the hand edema?

    A. Compression wrapping
    B. Positional elevation
    C. Retrograde massage
    D. PROM exercises

49. A client who has recently been diagnosed with fibromyalgia reports that hand pain and stiffness make it difficult to grasp a standard knife and fork during mealtimes. Which assistive devices should the OTR **INITIALLY** recommend for this client?

    A. Utensils with built-up handles
    B. Rocker knife and plate with raised sides
    C. Universal cuff with wrist support
    D. Lightweight utensils with non-slip grips

50. An OTR is using proprioceptive neuromuscular facilitation during functional activities with a client who has Stage 2 Parkinson's disease. Which of the following techniques would be included as part of the intervention with this client?

    A. Rhythmic initiation
    B. Fast brushing
    C. Joint approximation
    D. Reciprocal Inhibition

51. An OTR is fabricating a static splint for a partial thickness burn to the dorsum of the hand. The primary purpose of the splint is to maintain the length of the MCP joint collateral ligaments. To achieve this goal, the splint should be fabricated to position the MCP joints, IP joints, and wrist in which of the following positions?

	MCP Joint Position	IP Joint Position	Wrist Positions
A.	20° - 30° flexion	20° - 25° flexion	25° - 30° extension
B.	35° - 45° flexion	30° - 40° flexion	neutral
C.	fully extended	45° - 60° flexion	neutral
D.	60° - 70° flexion	0° - 5° flexion	25° - 30° extension

52. An OTR who works in an outpatient clinic is evaluating a client who was referred for a splint. The OTR notes a claw-hand deformity of the involved hand. Which type of splint is indicated for this client?

  A. Dorsal-based MCP joint blocking splint with a dynamic component to pull the ring and small finger IP joints into extension
  B. Low-profile dynamic splint that blocks hyperextension of digits 2-5, and has an IP join extension outrigger
  C. Forearm and hand volar-based static splint to block MCP joint hyperextension, but allow active IP joint motion
  D. Hand-based static splint that blocks the MCP joints of digits 4-5 in flexion, but allows IP joint motion

53. A 5-year-old child sustained partial and full thickness burns on the volar surfaces of both wrists and forearms three months ago. The child now wears pressure garments, but still has thick scars that are beginning to limit wrist mobility. One of the intervention objectives is to maximize wrist motion. Which activity would be **MOST EFFECTIVE** for progressing toward this goal?

  A. Tossing bean bags at a target
  B. Playing parachute games with peers
  C. Bouncing a medium-size therapy ball
  D. Creeping through a play tunnel maze

54. Which of the following symptoms are **TYPICALLY** indications that a client who has been on prolonged bed rest is experiencing orthostatic hypotension?

  A. Diaphoresis when turning over from supine to side-lying position
  B. Lightheadedness upon moving from a supine to seated position
  C. Shortness of breath when sitting up from a supine position
  D. Pounding headache upon moving into a semi-reclined position

Sample Items

55. An OTR is completing a home visit for a client who had a total hip replacement 2 weeks ago. What type of seat should the OTR recommend the client use when sitting at home to watch television?

   A. Firm raised chair with a wedge cushion insert and armrests
   B. Cushioned, armless dining chair elevated on one inch-blocks
   C. Sofa with pillows for lateral trunk support
   D. Overstuffed reclining chair with pillows to elevate the leg in extension

56. A patient who had a myocardial infarction 2 days ago is beginning phase I of cardiac rehabilitation. Which of the following actions is **ESSENTIAL** for the OTR to do during the client's initial session?

   A. Provide instruction on stress management.
   B. Monitor the client's orthostatic tolerance.
   C. Initiate reconditioning and isometric activities.
   D. Teach the client to measure energy expenditure.

57. A client with rheumatoid arthritis should use which of the following joint protection techniques when completing kitchen tasks?

   A. Grasping cookware with the fingertips
   B. Transporting items using a wheeled cart
   C. Using weighted utensils during meal preparation
   D. Twisting a jar lid open with the right hand

58. An OTR is evaluating a client who fractured the right dominant wrist six weeks ago and had the short arm cast removed one day ago. The client holds the affected arm in a guarded position and rates the pain as 6/10 on a visual analog scale. There is moderate pitting edema of the hand and forearm. The client is able to flex the fingers to within three fingers-breadth of the palm. Which of the following should be included as part of this client's **INITIAL** intervention plan?

   A. Dynamic finger flexion splinting
   B. Passive ROM exercises
   C. Manual edema mobilization
   D. Gentle stress loading exercises

59. A patient is recovering from partial and full thickness burns on the dominant upper extremity has recently developed heterotopic ossification (HO) at the elbow. Prior to the onset of the HO, the patient was independent with self-feeding. Now, the patient tends to use only the non-dominant hand due to symptoms associated with the HO. Which of the following assistive devices would be **MOST BENEFICIAL** for this patient?

   A. Universal cuff with elongated utensil
   B. Swivel spoon and elongated utensils
   C. Rocker knife with a built-up handle
   D. Mechanical feeder with supinator attachment

60. A client who has a lesion of the cerebellum is participating in OT to increase independence with self-feeding. Which assistive devices should the client use to promote progress toward this goal?

    A. Suction plate and cup holder
    B. Side-cutting fork and rocker knife
    C. Plastic cup and lightweight utensils
    D. Universal cuff with mobile arm support

61. Which of the following environmental adaptations will improve safety during meal preparation for a client who has low vision?

    A. Installing a microwave that has preprogrammed cooking options
    B. Placing tactile markings on the operating knobs of the appliances
    C. Arranging items on the pantry and cabinet shelves in alphabetical order
    D. Use large-sized bowls and pots for mixing and stove-top cooking

62. An inpatient who has hemiparesis is preparing for discharge from a rehabilitation unit to home. The patient uses a wheelchair for mobility and completes self-care independently using assistive devices. The patient's home is equipped with a standard bathtub, and a separate walk-in shower that has a safety glass door with a 6-inch high doorsill. Both the shower and the tub have safety grab bars. Which piece of durable medical equipment would be **MOST BENEFICIAL** for this patient to use at home?

    A. Padded transfer bench with swivel seat for the bathtub
    B. Shower chair that can be used in the shower or bathtub
    C. Plastic bath chair with armrests and accessory caddy
    D. Transfer board and plastic shower stool with a contoured seat

63. A mobile arm support is **CONTRAINDICATED** to recommend for clients who have which of the following diagnoses?

    A. Incomplete C_4 spinal cord injury
    B. Guillain-Barré syndrome
    C. Huntington's disease
    D. Amyotrophic lateral sclerosis

64. An OTR is teaching stand-pivot transfers to a client who has Stage 2 Parkinson's disease and uses a wheelchair for mobility. After instructing the client to properly position the chair in relation to the transfer surface, and asking the client to lock the wheelchair brakes, what should the OTR ask the client to do **NEXT**?

    A. Scoot the hips forward to the edge of the wheelchair.
    B. Come to standing by pushing up on the wheelchair arm rests.
    C. Rock forward while reaching toward the transfer surface.
    D. Position both feet perpendicular to the transfer surface.

65. Which activity represents an effective sensory integrative approach for improving tolerance to touch for a 5-year-old child who has mild tactile defensiveness?

A. Swinging in a prone position in a net swing
B. Spinning in a seated position on a scooter board
C. Using a feather boa while playing dress-up activity
D. Log rolling to wrap tightly in a blanket

66. What is the **MOST EFFECTIVE** method for grading an activity to improve muscular endurance?

A. Maintaining the same resistance and increasing the number of repetitions
B. Shortening the interval of time to complete a controlled set of isotonic exercises
C. Increasing resistance to 75% of maximal strength and maintaining repetitions
D. Decreasing repetitions and increasing resistance for short intervals of time

67. A client who has multiple sclerosis has recently transitioned from assisted ambulation to using a standard wheelchair for mobility. A recent onset of fatigue, upper extremity weakness, and back and neck discomfort is beginning to interfere with job performance. The client is employed as a magazine editor, and spends much of the day sitting in the wheelchair while working at the computer monitor positioned at eye level. The client wants to continue sitting in a wheelchair to avoid having to complete transfers when moving from the desk to other parts of the work area. Which modification would be **MOST BENEFICIAL** for this client?

A. Power scooter with padded seat and electric tilt-in-space control
B. Voice-controlled computer system and telephone headset
C. Solid seat insert, lumbar support and bilateral forearm supports
D. Deltoid aid and a split design computer keyboard

68. An inpatient who has borderline personality disorder has been hospitalized due to an exacerbation of suicidal and self-mutilating behavior. An initial evaluation indicates the patient is functioning at Allen Cognitive Level V (Exploratory actions). The patient reports being overwhelmed by a new personal relationship, experiencing job dissatisfaction, and feeling a lack of control in many daily situations. Which intervention activity would be **MOST BENEFICIAL** for this patient?

A. Coping skills groups that address a variety of adaptive strategies
B. One-on-one sessions to encourage the patient to contract for safety
C. Daily self-care sessions that focus on structured BADL
D. Structured one-step craft activities to promote successful outcomes

69. A young adult who has chronic schizophrenia and is functioning at Allen Cognitive Level 4 (Goal-directed Actions) is able to wash clothes independently in a washing machine operated with push-button settings. When the machine is replaced with one that has a dial setting, the client is unable to use the new machine correctly. Which compensatory techniques would be **MOST EFFECTIVE** to improve this client's ability to use the new machine?

    A. Provide the client with verbal cueing to learn the task.
    B. Teach the client to use mnemonics for operating the machine.
    C. Display step-by-step illustrated directions next to the machine.
    D. Encourage a trial-and-error approach for learning the new sequence.

70. An 8-year-old child sustained second-degree burn to the first web space of both hands one month ago. Re-evaluation shows that the child's web space is contracting; despite wearing pressure garments, using splints at night, and completing home program activities. Which intervention would be **MOST EFFECTIVE** based on these findings?

    A. Advise the caregiver to increase the intensity and frequency of passive ROM exercises.
    B. Begin serial splinting that incorporates a polymer gel sheet over the affected areas.
    C. Provide the caregiver with a list of age-appropriate games that will promote hand use.
    D. Use a paraffin modality during OT sessions to soften the scar prior to functional activity.

71. An individual who has had a TBI and is functioning at Level VII (Automatic-appropriate) on the Rancho Los Amigos scale is participating in OT. The individual currently has a maximum attention span of 15 minutes and is able to follow two-step commands. The individual plans to return home to resume homemaking roles. One of the individual's short-term goals is to bake cookies for a family member's upcoming birthday. How should the activity be graded to promote the successful accomplishment of this goal?

    A. Have the individual prepare cookies using slice and bake ready-made cookie dough.
    B. Provide the individual with a detailed recipe to bake cookies from scratch.
    C. Have the individual prepare cookies using a boxed cookie mix with pre-measured dry ingredients.
    D. Mix the ingredients together and have the individual drop the cookies onto a pan.

72. A client who is legally blind reports having difficulty locating grooming items in the bathroom every morning, resulting in being late for work. Which recommendation should the OTR suggest for improving this client's occupational performance?

    A. Complete the majority of bathing and grooming tasks the night before.
    B. Wake-up at least one hour earlier so that grooming will not be rushed.
    C. Arrange items in the bathroom so that there is a specific place for each item.
    D. Discuss with the employer options for implementing a later start time at work.

73. An OTR plans to use a sensorimotor approach to improve handwriting skills of a 6-year-old student who has a mild learning disability. The student maintains a very tight grip on a pencil when writing, consistently uses a palmar grasp when holding the pencil, and has directional confusion when forming letters. Which activity represents this approach and would be effective to include as part of the **INITIAL** intervention?

A. Painting letters using a wide-barrel brush on paper attached to an upright easel
B. Rolling out colored modeling dough and making cookie cutter shapes on a tabletop
C. Using spring-opening blunt-edge scissors to cut out geometric paper shapes
D. Providing hand-over-hand assistance during writing assignments

74. A 12-month-old child has moderate hypotonia resulting in developmental delay and poor oral motor control. Which position is recommend for this child for promoting oral motor function during feeding?

A. Slightly reclined with trunk fully supported and the neck and head at midline
B. Fully upright in sitting with the head and neck resting in slight extension
C. Seated upright in a standard high with a lap tray in positioned close to the chest
D. Semi-reclined in a position of comfort on a soft beanbag chair

75. A client is recovering from a recent acute exacerbation of multiple sclerosis. The client becomes moderately fatigued during lower extremity dressing the morning after beginning an upgraded exercise program the prior afternoon. The client denies other changes in the activity patterns over the past several days. Which action should the OTR take with regards to the intervention activities for the **NEXT** day?

A. Maintain the current exercise level and monitor symptoms.
B. Eliminate the exercises and continue with the ADL plans.
C. Reduce the intensity of the exercises to the previous level.
D. Have the client focus on upper extremity dressing in sitting.

76. A school-based OTR is selecting seating alternatives for a student who has moderate hypotonia and has just transitioned to a full-day kindergarten program. The student uses a wheelchair for mobility and does not tolerate an upright sitting position throughout the school day. What type of positioning system is **MOST BENEFICIAL** for this student?

A. Lightweight chair with reclining back and reverse wheel configuration
B. Corner chair with high lateral supports that can be placed on the floor
C. Dense foam lateral supports and gel cushion for the current wheelchair
D. Modular wheelchair with tilt-in-space feature in the mobility base

77. A client who has been hospitalized with the early stages of a slow, progressive upper motor neuron disease has been on a leave of absence from a job as an accountant. The client now ambulates with a cane, uses a wheelchair for distance mobility, has mild intention tremors, and fatigues quickly. Which of the following is considered a reasonable accommodation that the employer is required to provide to this employee?

A. Consideration for modifying the client's current work schedule
B. Employee review to change the essential elements of the job description
C. Provision of a wheelchair at the job site in case of emergency
D. Modification of doorways throughout the workplace for maximal accessibility

78. An OTR is implementing a leisure education program for clients who participate in an outpatient chemical dependency program. Which data is **MOST BENEFICIAL** to use for measuring the effectiveness of the program?

A. Amount of family and community support for client before entering the program and upon completion of the program
B. Number of clients pursuing leisure interests before and after completing the program
C. Self-assessment questionnaire the clients fill out during the last session
D. Frequency of contact between staff and client during the program

79. An inpatient who has had a TBI is functioning at Level V (Confused-inappropriate) on the Rancho Los Amigos scale. Which of the following approaches would an OTR use to facilitate the patient's success during a grooming task?

A. Provide repeated verbal instructions until the patient completes the task.
B. Use forward chaining techniques if the patient is distracted from the task.
C. Demonstrate a portion of the activity then ask the patient return demonstration.
D. Give one-step instructions and hand-over-hand cueing throughout the task.

80. A client who had a CVA one month ago now has moderate-severe flexor spasticity and scapular immobility of the involved upper extremity. Which technique is **CONTRAINDICATED** to use for minimizing the impact of the spasticity on passive mobility for dressing and hygiene?

A. Self-ROM exercises in supine several times per day
B. Reciprocal pulley exercises using wall mounted pulleys
C. Upper extremity weight-bearing during functional tasks
D. Long-arm air splinting prior to completing a self-care task

81. An inpatient who has COPD begins to have dyspnea when putting on a pair of pants while seated on a bedside chair during a dressing session. Pulse oximetry indicates that the patient's oxygen saturation is at 93%. After stopping the activity, what should the OTR have the patient do **NEXT**?

   A. Take several shallow breaths through the mouth.
   B. Breathe in through the nose and slowly exhale.
   C. Inhale through the mouth and quickly exhale.
   D. Begin wearing an oxygen nasal cannula.

82. An OTR is developing an intervention plan for an inpatient who has severe post-traumatic stress disorder. Symptoms started several weeks after being robbed in a convenience store where the patient was working. The patient's goal is to resume work at the store, but extreme fear and distrust interfere with the ability to interact with customers. Which context is **MOST** conducive for promoting initial progress toward a return-to-work goal with this patient?

   A. One-on-one in the patient's room
   B. During a group role-play session
   C. In the hospital gift shop
   D. In a discussion group with several other patients

83. An OTR is working with a patient who recently had a complete T_5 spinal cord injury and has been in the intensive care unit on extended bed-rest. The patient has been able to sit in bed without dizziness with the head of the bed elevated to 45° for one-hour intervals. Which position is safest for the patient to be placed in **NEXT**?

   A. Upright in a standard wheelchair with close monitoring
   B. Upright on a tilt-table at 90° while wearing an abdominal binder and elastic stockings
   C. Seated in a semi-reclining reclining wheelchair with legs elevated
   D. Seated on the edge of the bed with both legs unsupported and knees flexed to 90°

84. An OTR is working with the caregiver of a client who has Stage II Alzheimer's disease. The caregiver reports that the client wanders throughout the home at night to use the bathroom, and occasionally has walked out the front door instead of into the bathroom. Which environmental adaptation should the OTR recommend to the caregiver?

   A. Using movement sensitive audio-visual assistive technology
   B. Placing a commode chair in the client's bedroom
   C. Installing a video monitor in several locations in the house
   D. Keeping hallway and bedroom lights on at night

Uphold professional standards and responsibilities to promote quality in practice

85. An OTR who works in a skilled nursing facility frequently provides residents with adaptive devices to improve functional performance. Which of the following methods is **MOST EFFECTIVE** for evaluating the impact of an adaptive device for supporting the residents' participation in occupation?

   A. Tracking the number of times the client brings the device to OT sessions
   B. Having the client verbalize understanding of the functional use of the device
   C. Ask the client to demonstrate the use of the device for a specific activity
   D. Observing the client spontaneously using the device for a variety of activities

86. A client who had a finger fracture secondary to an athletic injury 8 weeks ago now has a finger PIP joint contracture. The OTR has just fabricated a dynamic extension splint as per the physician's request. Which information is **MOST IMPORTANT** for the OTR to include in the client contact note?

   A. Results of a sensory evaluation of the affected hand
   B. Goniometric measurements of the affected hand
   C. Thickness and type of material used for the splint
   D. Splint construction methods and care instructions

87. An OTR who works in a pediatric hospital-based clinic wants to begin using a newly developed listening device as part of the OT intervention for children who have autism. What ethical responsibility does the OTR have prior to integrating the use of this device into intervention plans?

   A. Outline a standard protocol to use with each child who will use the device.
   B. Identify the institutional policies and clinical evidence about using the device.
   C. Develop a plan to monitor the effectiveness of the new intervention.
   D. Determine if third-party payers reimburse the device as a therapeutic modality.

88. An individual worked as an OTR in an outpatient setting for four years, but has not been employed as an OT or pursued continuing education in OT for the past 6 years. The individual wants to resume OT clinical practice in an outpatient setting. Which of the following tasks should the individual **INITIALLY** complete in pursuit of this goal?

   A. Identify the professional development units that can be carried over from the previous job.
   B. Work as a volunteer OT practitioner in the desired setting until service competency is established.
   C. Identify an effective learning plan related to practice skills needed for the desired job.
   D. Submit applications for certification renewal and state licensure.

SECTION 5

Sample Items

89. Which of the following situations represents a potential violation of the ethical principle related to "Dual Relationships" by an OT fieldwork supervisor?

    A. Attending the OT graduation of a former fieldwork level II supervisee
    B. Agreeing to meet a fieldwork level II student at a coffee shop after work to discuss a thesis topic
    C. Leading a study group after work hours in the OT clinic for OT and OTA students
    D. Speaking to the academic fieldwork supervisor about a fieldwork student without the student's permission

90. A fieldwork level II student is evaluating a client in an outpatient setting. The supervising OTR observes that the student is altering the administrative procedures outlined in the standardized testing manual. Which statement represents the type of timely feedback that the supervisor should provide to the student?

    A. "Can you tell me your reasons for using the tool in this manner?"
    B. "Why are you using the incorrect procedures for administering this test?"
    C. "I like that you are using this test, but you must follow the correct procedures."
    D. "You need to stop the test and review the testing manual more thoroughly."

91. An OTR who works on the adolescent unit of an inpatient psychiatric facility observes that an OT fieldwork student has been showing signs of burnout. During a team meeting, one of the team members voiced a complaint about the OT services that the student has been providing. What **INITIAL** action should the OTR take regarding the student's performance at work?

    A. Document the complaint and observations in the student's fieldwork record.
    B. Talk with the student to obtain pertinent facts surrounding the issues.
    C. Meet with the academic fieldwork coordinator to discuss the student.
    D. Provide the student with practical solutions for avoiding burnout.

92. An OTR is planning to give a presentation to a support group for individuals who have recently been diagnosed with multiple sclerosis. The group wants to learn about the role of occupational therapy in the management of this disease process. Which information should be included in the presentation to **MOST EFFECTIVELY** address this topic?

    A. A description of the various types of assessments used when providing OT
    B. A discussion about OT for maintaining health and preventing dysfunction
    C. A demonstration of an OT session using a group participant as an example
    D. An outline of OT protocols typically used for individuals who have this disease

93. An OTR is writing a letter to an insurance company appealing the company's denial for reimbursement of pre-authorized OT services. What information related to the client is **MOST IMPORTANT** to include in this letter?

   A. An outline of functional tasks used during each intervention session
   B. A summary of progress with reference to the initial evaluation and functional goals
   C. An annotated reference list indicating evidence related to best practice guidelines
   D. The rate of progress compared to other individuals who have the same diagnosis

94. An individual who has had a recent bilateral below knee amputation is an inpatient in a Medicare funded rehabilitation facility. The individual participates in 3 hours of therapy per day, and is currently scheduled for discharge in two weeks. At the weekly interdisciplinary meeting, the OTR reports that the patient has met all intervention goals. The physical therapist anticipates that the patient will require physical therapy sessions 2 hours per day for the full 2 weeks of therapy to meet specified physical therapy goals. What action should the OTR take based on this meeting?

   A. Complete a discharge summary and discontinue the patient from OT services.
   B. Determine if there are any other activities in which the patient would like to participate.
   C. Schedule the patient for at least one hour of OT per day to meet the three-hour therapy rule.
   D. Continue to schedule OT sessions to maintain the progress that the patient has made thus far.

95. Two weeks away from completing a level II fieldwork placement at an acute inpatient rehabilitation facility, an OT student's onsite fieldwork supervisor sustains an injury and is unable to work for 6 weeks. Of the following individuals, who should provide supervision to the student for the remainder of the placement?

   A. An OTR who has a faculty appointment from the student's academic program.
   B. A licensed and certified OTA who has worked at the facility for 5 years.
   C. A newly certified contract OTR who is taking over the fieldwork supervisor's caseload.
   D. A licensed rehabilitation professional in the department who has trans-disciplinary training.

96. A patient, who has had a CVA resulting in global aphasia and flaccid hemiplegia, has been making slow progress in OT. During a non-patient care in-service, a co-worker, who is the patient's distant relative, asks about the patient's progress. Which statement represents an appropriate response for the OTR to provide?

   A. "Based on the recent evaluation, the patient has a long way to go."
   B. "I can't talk about the patient without the patient's approval."
   C. "The patient seems to be satisfied with the overall progress."
   D. "I think the patient will have a hard time returning home."

97. Which of the following **MUST** an OTR include as part of the NBCOT certification renewal application process?

    A. Attestation related to the Certificant Code of Conduct
    B. Evidence of completing Professional Development Units
    C. Proof of membership in the professional association
    D. An updated professional development plan

98. An OTR has completed the initial evaluation of an inpatient who has cancer. The OTR plans to work with the patient on a daily basis prior to the patient's planned discharge to home in one week. What information is **MOST IMPORTANT** to include in the initial evaluation report?

    A. Summary data as it relates to the occupational profile
    B. Details about interventions for promoting goal attainment
    C. Descriptions of community support services available
    D. Recommendations for post-discharge OT services

99. A rheumatologist has prescribed bilateral nighttime resting hand splints for a child who has early stage juvenile rheumatoid arthritis. The parents ask the OTR who works at the child's school to fabricate the splints. Despite having this disease, the child is functioning at grade-level and is not on the OT caseload. What action should the OTR take in response to the parents' request?

    A. Schedule a time after school hours to fabricate the splints for the child.
    B. Initiate an IEP indicating the child's needs for school-based OT.
    C. Inform the parents to schedule an appointment at an outpatient OT clinic.
    D. Provide the parents with catalog information for ordering pre-fabricated splints.

100. An OTR is conducting a literature search about the effectiveness of using a inhibitory technique prior to a functional activity for reducing muscle tone in patients who have spastic hemiplegia. Findings from one of the articles indicate a 0.09 probability that this intervention is effective while another article has a p-value of 0.04. How should the OTR **INITIALLY** proceed in interpreting these findings from a clinical perspective?

    A. Conclude that the evidence-based research does not support the use of this intervention.
    B. Determine if there is additional evidence-based research supporting the use of another type of modality.
    C. Recognize that the findings are conflicting and cannot be used to make clinical decisions.
    D. Identify the sample size differences between the two studies before making definitive conclusions.

Multiple-Choice Items

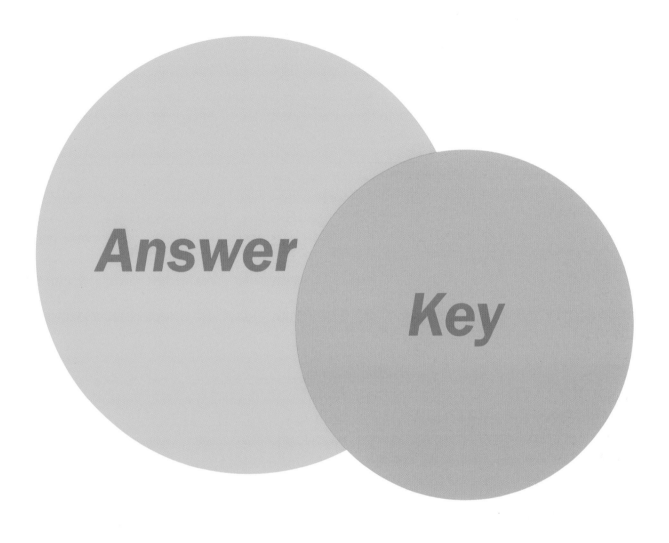

1-B	26-C	51-D	76-D
2-B	27-D	52-D	77-A
3-A	28-D	53-D	78-B
4-A	29-A	54-B	79-D
5-D	30-A	55-A	80-B
6-C	31-D	56-B	81-B
7-A	32-C	57-B	82-A
8-D	33-C	58-C	83-C
9-C	34-B	59-B	84-A
10-B	35-D	60-A	85-D
11-D	36-A	61-B	86-B
12-B	37-B	62-A	87-B
13-A	38-C	63-C	88-C
14-D	39-A	64-A	89-B
15-B	40-C	65-D	90-A
16-D	41-B	66-A	91-B
17-D	42-D	67-C	92-B
18-C	43-A	68-A	93-B
19-A	44-C	69-C	94-A
20-A	45-C	70-B	95-A
21-B	46-C	71-A	96-B
22-A	47-B	72-C	97-A
23-C	48-B	73-A	98-A
24-B	49-A	74-A	99-C
25-B	50-A	75-C	100-D

1. *Correct Answer: B*

   Figure-ground perception is the ability to distinguish a foreground from the background. A child who has figure-ground deficits would have difficulty finding a specific size/shape bead in a bag of beads.

   Incorrect Answers:

   A, C, D: Figure-ground deficits would not be as evident during these activities.

   Reference: Zoltan, B. (2007). *Vision, Perception, and Cognition: A Manual for the Evaluation and Treatment of the Adult with Acquired Brain Injury* (4th ed.). Thorofare, NJ: SLACK Inc. Pages 155-159.

2. *Correct Answer: B*

   This skill requires a complex integration of visual and somatosensory systems that typically develops by the third year of age.

   Incorrect Answers:

   A, C, D: These self-dressing skills typically develop prior to age three.

   Reference: Case-Smith, J. (2005). *Occupational Therapy for Children* (5th ed.). St. Louis, MO: Elsevier Mosby, Inc. Page 547.

3. *Correct Answer: A*

   An understanding of the contexts that impact a child's performance is critical to effective intervention planning.

   Incorrect Answers:

   B, C, D: This information is helpful but is not a critical component for OT intervention planning.

   Reference: Case-Smith, J. (2005). *Occupational Therapy for Children* (5th ed.). St. Louis, MO: Elsevier Mosby, Inc. Pages 219-220.

4. *Correct Answer: A*

   This is a survey used as a measure of general health and well-being. It has been used in medical outcomes studies and is sensitive to change in health status.

   Incorrect Answers:

   B: This is an evaluation of basic living skills and does not measure quality of life.

   C: This is an evaluation for assessing severity of a disability and does not measure quality of life.

   D: This reflects the functional status of hospital patients. It is not a measure of quality of life.

   Reference: Asher IE. (2007). *Occupational Therapy Assessment Tool: An Annotated Index.* (3rd ed.). Bethesda, MD: AOTA Press. Pages 64, 80, 102, 224.

SECTION 5

Sample Items

5. *Correct Answer: D*

This fosters collaboration between the client and OTR for developing a meaningful client-centered intervention plan. It can be used to measure change in a client's self-perception of occupational performance over time.

Incorrect Answers:

A: This is an evaluation of basic living skills and does not address the client's priorities.

B: This reflects the functional status of hospital patients and does not address the client's priorities.

C: This helps to identify roles significant to the client and the motivation to engage in the tasks necessary for those roles.

Reference: Asher IE. (2007). *Occupational Therapy Assessment Tool: An Annotated Index* (3rd ed.). Bethesda, MD: AOTA Press. Pages 33, 80, 102, 627.

6. *Correct Answer: C*

Task performance is influenced by environmental surroundings. Therefore, it is best for the work readiness tasks to take place in the actual work environment.

Incorrect Answers:

A, B, D: These contexts are helpful when observing a client perform a cooking task, but these are not the **BEST** contexts for determining the influence of environmental demands on the client's task performance.

Reference: Pendleton HM, Schultz-Krohn W (eds). (2006). *Pedretti's Occupational Therapy: Practice Skills for Physical Dysfunction* (6th ed.). St. Louis: Elsevier Mosby. Page 9.

7. *Correct Answer: A*

Ecology of human performance (EHP) model focuses on tasks that acquire meaning through the person-environment interaction. Modifying the client's home environment will enhance the client's well-being and quality of life in that environment.

Incorrect Answers:

B, C, D: These do not support the EHP approach.

Reference: Radomski, M. V. & Trombly-Latham, C. (2008). *Occupational Therapy for Physical Dysfunction* (6th ed.). Baltimore, MD: Walters Kluwer, Lippincott, Williams & Wilkins. Pages 286.

8. *Correct Answer: D*

This is a functionally based approach for clients who have had a CVA.

Incorrect Answers:

A: This is a bottom-up approach based on a neurophysiological model.

B: This uses a bottom-up approach that aims to inhibit abnormal reflex mechanisms to facilitate function.

C: This uses a top-down approach of adapting a client's environment to compensate for symptoms.

Reference: Zoltan B. (2007). *Vision, Perception, and Cognition: A Manual for the Evaluation and Treatment of the Adult with Acquired Brain Injury* (4th ed.). Thorofare, NJ: SLACK, Inc. Page 9.

9. *Correct Answer: C*

The assessment should take place in the environment where the individual will typically complete this task. While an inpatient, this is in the bathroom of the patient's room.

Incorrect Answers:

A, B, D: These are not optimal environments for completing this assessment.

Reference: Radomski, M. V. & Trombly-Latham, C. (2008). *Occupational Therapy for Physical Dysfunction* (6th ed.). Baltimore, MD: Walters Kluwer, Lippincott, Williams & Wilkins. Pages 80-82.

10. *Correct Answer: B*

The radial nerve is commonly injured with a fracture of the humerus. This results in weak or absent wrist and finger extensors. The OTR should contact the physician to verify the radial nerve palsy and to clarify the consult before proceeding with rehabilitation for the hand.

Incorrect Answers:

A: This is not indicated in the presence of radial nerve palsy.

C: These may be appropriate after determining if a radial nerve palsy is present and upon clarification of the therapy consult.

D: Manual muscle testing is not indicated in the presence of a healing fracture.

Reference: Burke S, Higgins J, McClinton M, Saunders R, Valdata L. (2006). *Hand and Upper Extremity Rehabilitation: A Practical Guide* (3rd ed.). St. Louis: Elsevier Churchill Livingstone. Page 337.

Pendleton HM, Schultz-Krohn W (eds). (2006). *Pedretti's Occupational Therapy: Practice Skills for Physical Dysfunction* (6th ed.). St. Louis: Elsevier Mosby. Pages 994-995.

11. *Correct Answer: D*

Occupational profiles provide information about the client's priorities. This leads to a more individualized approach to evaluation and intervention planning.

Incorrect Answers:

A, B, C: These may be helpful during the evaluation process, but only after completion of a comprehensive occupational profile.

Reference: Radomski, M. V. & Trombly-Latham, C. (2008). *Occupational Therapy for Physical Dysfunction* (6th ed.). Baltimore, MD: Walters Kluwer, Lippincott, Williams & Wilkins. Pages 1181-1182.

12. *Correct Answer: B*

The adaptive approach capitalizes on the client's abilities. This top-down approach aims to facilitate functional performance through compensatory techniques.

Incorrect Answers:

A, C, D: These are examples of a restorative approach.

Reference: Zoltan, B. (2007). *Vision, Perception, and Cognition: A Manual for the Evaluation and Treatment of the Adult with Acquired Brain Injury* (4th ed.). Thorofare, NJ: SLACK, Inc. Pages 4-5, 100-103.

13. *Correct Answer: A*

This answer supports a client-centered, collaborative approach.

Incorrect Answers:

B: Assistive devices are not essential for the patient to use.

C: Using assistive devices does not necessarily speed up the healing process.

D: The OTR should talk with the patient and patient's spouse prior to documenting an impression or contacting a care coordinator.

Reference: Radomski, M. V. & Trombly-Latham, C. (2008). *Occupational Therapy for Physical Dysfunction* (6th ed.). Baltimore, MD: Walters Kluwer, Lippincott, Williams & Wilkins. Pages 311-312.

14. *Correct Answer: D*

This approach is client-centered and emphasizes the environment as a facilitator and barrier of occupational performance during valued tasks.

Incorrect Answers:

A, B, C: These do not support an ecological model.

Reference: Radomski, M. V. & Trombly-Latham, C. (2008). *Occupational Therapy for Physical Dysfunction* (6th ed.). Baltimore, MD: Walters Kluwer, Lippincott, Williams & Wilkins. Page 286.

15. *Correct Answer: B*

Individuals who have constructional apraxia have difficulty constructing/assembling objects; as in preparing a sandwich.

Incorrect Answers:

A, C, D: These tasks do not require assembly or construction of objects.

Reference: Zoltan, B. (2007). *Vision, Perception, and Cognition: A Manual for the Evaluation and Treatment of the Adult with Acquired Brain Injury* (4th ed.). Thorofare, NJ: SLACK, Inc. Pages 123-128, 184.

16. *Correct Answer: D*

A client functioning at this level has localized responses to some stimuli. It is important to establish an objective baseline of responsiveness.

Incorrect Answers:

A, B, C: These are not appropriate for a client who is functioning at Level III (Localized response).

Reference: Radomski, M. V. & Trombly-Latham, C. (2008). *Occupational Therapy for Physical Dysfunction* (6th ed.). Baltimore, MD: Walters Kluwer, Lippincott, Williams & Wilkins. Pages 1059-1060.

17. *Correct Answer: D*

The radial wrist extensors typically are innervated in individuals who have a complete C_6 spinal cord injury. This allows individuals to use a tenodesis grasp to attain a higher level of functional independence.

Incorrect Answers:

A: Finger and thumb flexors are innervated at the C_7 level.

B: Elbow extension is innervated at the C_7 level and is not present in a complete C_6 spinal cord injury.

C: Trunk control for side bending is absent at the C_5-C_6 level.

Reference: Radomski, M. V. & Trombly-Latham, C. (2008). *Occupational Therapy for Physical Dysfunction* (6th ed.). Baltimore, MD: Walters Kluwer, Lippincott, Williams & Wilkins. Pages 1188-1190.

18. *Correct Answer: C*

Volumetric measurement procedures are standardized and would produce the **MOST RELIABLE** results for measuring hand edema for clients with this diagnosis.

Incorrect Answers:

A, B, D: These can be useful for measuring edema, but typically the procedures for each are not completed using standardized methods.

Reference: Gillen, G., Burkhardt, A. (2004). *Stroke Rehabilitation: A Function-Based Approach* (2nd ed.). St. Louis: Mosby. Pages: 222-223.

Pendleton, H.M., Schultz-Krohn, W. (eds). (2006). *Pedretti's Occupational Therapy: Practice Skills for Physical Dysfunction* (6th ed.). St. Louis, MO: Elsevier Mosby. Pages 171-172.

19. *Correct Answer: A*

Since the patient has intact memory, the behavior suggests topographical disorientation. The test for this is typically a functional test.   Contributing visual perceptual deficits should also be considered.

Incorrect Answers:

B, C, D: The client's behaviors are not consistent with deficits in these areas.

Reference: Zoltan, B. (2007). *Vision, Perception, and Cognition: A Manual for the Evaluation and Treatment of the Adult with Acquired Brain Injury* (4th ed.).   Thorofare, NJ: SLACK, Inc. Page 165.

20. *Correct Answer: A*

Visual foundation skills include visual acuity, visual fields, and oculomotor control. The OTR should base plans for completing a standardized perceptual test only after a screening of the patient's pre-morbid visual foundation skills.

Incorrect Answers:

B, C, D: These will no impact the accuracy of a visual perceptual assessment.

Reference: Radomski, M. V. & Trombly-Latham, C. (2008). *Occupational Therapy for Physical Dysfunction* (6th ed.). Baltimore, MD: Walters Kluwer, Lippincott, Williams & Wilkins. Page 238.

Sample Items

21. *Correct Answer: B*

Ulnar nerve palsy at the wrist impairs the adductor pollicis muscle resulting in the inability to perform a "key" or lateral pinch.

Incorrect Answers:

A: Carrying a briefcase requires a hook grasp which is not affected by a low ulnar nerve injury.

C: This would be less evident when using the index finger to input numbers in a calculator. The lumbrical muscles flex the index finger MCP joint and are innervated by the median nerve.

D: Holding coins in the palm of the hand is not reliant upon an intact ulnar nerve.

Reference: Cooper, C. (2007). *Fundamentals of Hand Therapy: Clinical Reasoning and Treatment Guidelines for Common Diagnoses of the Upper Extremity.* St. Louis, MO: Elsevier Mosby. Page 237.

22. *Correct Answer: A*

This functional top-down approach involves compensation and adaptation to maximize a client's independence.

Incorrect Answers:

B, C, D: These are bottom-up restorative approaches.

Reference: Zoltan, B. (2007). *Vision, Perception, and Cognition: A Manual for the Evaluation and Treatment of the Adult with Acquired Brain Injury* (4th ed.). Thorofare, NJ: SLACK, Inc. Pages 16, 141.

23. *Correct Answer: C*

The concept of lifestyle redesign in the area of weight loss relies on occupational science research and theory. Emphasis is on improving quality of life by fostering meaningful engagement through healthful routines and activities.

Incorrect Answers:

A, B, D: These are not based primarily on the occupation science perspective.

Reference: Mandel, Jackson, Zemke, Nelson & Clark. (1999). *Implementing the Well Elderly Program.* MD: AOTA Press. Pages 11-17.

24. *Correct Answer: B*

Learning transfer techniques is important since the patient will require the caregivers to provide stand-by assistance.

Incorrect Answers:

A: This is not the role of the caregiver.

C: The patient should use energy conservation techniques during ADL, but these are not as important as transfer techniques for the caregiver to learn.

D: The patient should be able to complete this task without caregiver assistance.

Reference: Radomski, M. V. & Trombly-Latham, C. (2008). *Occupational Therapy for Physical Dysfunction* (6th ed.). Baltimore, MD: Walters Kluwer, Lippincott, Williams & Wilkins. Pages 1290-1291.

25. *Correct Answer:* B

The acquisition of practical life management skills is essential in enabling the client to develop a sense of control and autonomy for supporting participation in meaningful occupations.

Incorrect Answers:

A: Moving into an apartment with supportive friend, without establishing basic life management skills, leaves the client at risk for maladaptive behaviors, and other stressors.

C: Leisure activities with social acquaintances may not be effective if the social network includes individuals who are substance users.

D: The stem does not identify work stress as a current issue for this client.

Reference: Cara, E. & MacRae, A. (2005). *Psychosocial Occupational Therapy: A Clinical Practice* (2ⁿᵈ ed.). Thomson Delmar. Pages 447-469.

26. *Correct Answer:* C

The OTR should consult with the physician since splinting was not requested in the original consult.

Incorrect Answers:

A, B: These may be considered after consulting with the physician.

D: The OTR should not rely on the patient to initiate a referral.

Reference: Radomski, M. V. & Trombly-Latham, C. (2008). *Occupational Therapy for Physical Dysfunction* (6ᵗʰ ed.). Baltimore, MD: Walters Kluwer, Lippincott, Williams & Wilkins. 41-63.

27. *Correct Answer:* D

Limitations in active ROM, in the presence of full passive ROM, indicate weakness or a lack of power generated by the muscle or muscle group.

Incorrect Answers:

A: These are associated with ALS but would not cause this ROM discrepancy.

B, C: Active and passive ROM would be similarly impacted.

Reference: Radomski, M. V. & Trombly-Latham, C. (2008). *Occupational Therapy for Physical Dysfunction* (6ᵗʰ ed.). Baltimore, MD: Walters Kluwer, Lippincott, Williams & Wilkins. Pages 93, 124-126.

28. *Correct Answer:* D

The client has the right to refuse the use of the equipment, but in this case, the OTR can still work with the client to teach energy conservation and other compensatory techniques to promote the client's occupational performance.

Incorrect Answers:

A: The OTR should not coerce a client to use the equipment.

B: This is a potential violation of confidentiality

C: The OTR should respect the client's rights, but should not discharge the client from OT.

Reference: Radomski, M. V. & Trombly-Latham, C. (2008). *Occupational Therapy for Physical Dysfunction* (6ᵗʰ ed.). Baltimore, MD: Walters Kluwer, Lippincott, Williams & Wilkins. Pages 405-410, 412.

SECTION 5

Sample Items

29. *Correct Answer: A*

Axonotmesis typically resolves within 6 months without surgical intervention. Since sensation is impaired in the ulnar distribution, it is **MOST IMPORTANT** to teach the client to use visual skills as a compensatory means of protecting the hand from injury.

Incorrect Answers:

B: This is not indicated for this injury.

C: This can be initiated when Trace (1/5) muscle strength is evident.

D: This can be initiated as indicated when vibratory sensation is perceived.

Reference: Pendleton, H.M., Schultz-Krohn, W. (eds). (2006). *Pedretti's Occupational Therapy: Practice Skills for Physical Dysfunction* (6th ed.). St. Louis, MO: Elsevier Mosby. Pages 998-999.

30. *Correct Answer: A*

This movement pattern indicates the presence of the symmetrical tonic neck reflex (STNR).

Incorrect Answers:

B, C, D: These movement patterns are not consistent with the STNR.

Reference: Gentile, M. (2005). *Functional Visual Behavior in Children: A Guide to Evaluation and Treatment Options* (3rd ed.). Bethesda, MD: AOTA Press.   Pages 81-82.

31. *Correct Answer: D*

This is an appropriate goal for a patient who currently has non-specific, inconsistent, and non-purposeful reactions to stimuli.

Incorrect Answers:

A, B, C: These are goals for patients who are functioning at higher cognitive levels.

Reference: Radomski, M. V. & Trombly-Latham, C. (2008). *Occupational Therapy for Physical Dysfunction* (6th ed.). Baltimore, MD: Walters Kluwer, Lippincott, Williams & Wilkins. Pages 1050-1056.

32. *Correct Answer: C*

Identifying routines and habits is an essential element reestablishing a client's occupational functioning.

Incorrect Answers:

A, B, D: These can be done after determining a client's typical routines and habits.

Reference: Radomski, M. V. & Trombly-Latham, C. (2008). *Occupational Therapy for Physical Dysfunction* (6th ed.). Baltimore, MD: Walters Kluwer, Lippincott, Williams & Wilkins. Pages 50-56.

33. *Correct Answer: C*

The primary purpose of an interdisciplinary team approach is to make shared decisions and coordinate client care. Presenting this information to the team may support the goals of other team members. For example, nursing staff may be able to reinforce to the dining staff the need to properly position the patient for meals and to provide the patient with specific devices for feeding.

Incorrect Answers:

A: These are important to observe, but not important to report at a care coordination meeting.

B: Specific techniques do not need to be reported at a care coordination meeting.

D: Typically, patients who have dysphagia are provided with a special diet menu that consists of safe food options.

Reference: Radomski, M. V. & Trombly-Latham, C. (2008). *Occupational Therapy for Physical Dysfunction* (6ᵗʰ ed.). Baltimore, MD: Walters Kluwer, Lippincott, Williams & Wilkins. Page 1337.

34. *Correct Answer: B*

It is important to provide a structured environment with minimal distractions during the initial phase of intervention.

Incorrect Answers:

A: This may have negative effects on the client's ability to complete concrete tasks.

C, D: These do not provide the structure that the client needs at this stage of intervention.

Reference: Cara, E. & MacRae, A. (2005). *Psychosocial Occupational Therapy: A Clinical Practice* . (2ⁿᵈ ed.). Thomson Delmar. Pages 176-185.

35. *Correct Answer: D*

Goals and objectives are more likely to be successful if services are providing in the student's natural environment.

Incorrect Answers:

A, B, C: It may be helpful to occasionally provide the student an opportunity to practice a particular skill in these environments. However, it would not be as effective for the majority of the intervention sessions.

Reference: Case-Smith, J. (2005). *Occupational Therapy for Children* (5ᵗʰ ed.). St. Louis, MO: Elsevier Mosby, Inc. Page 814.

36. *Correct Answer: A*

The OTR should consult with the physician, as these are signs of clinical depression.

Incorrect Answers:

B: The OTR should not rely on the patient to initiate the appointment.

C, D: These may be considered after consulting with the physician.

Reference: Zoltan, B. (2007). *Vision, Perception, and Cognition: A Manual for the Evaluation and Treatment of the Adult with Acquired Brain Injury* (4ᵗʰ ed.). Thorofare, NJ: SLACK, Inc. Page 304.

Sample Items

37. *Correct Answer: B*

The percentile score is the percentage of subjects that score at or below a particular raw score.

Incorrect Answers:

A, C, D: These are not accurate statements based on the definition of a percentile score.

Reference: Case-Smith, J. (2005). *Occupational Therapy for Children* (5th ed.). St. Louis, MO: Elsevier Mosby, Inc. Page 257.

38. *Correct Answer: C*

The OTR should provide the client with opportunities to explore work habits and current abilities prior to selecting a specific employment placement.

Incorrect Answers:

A: This is a more appropriate option for individuals who have mental retardation, significant developmental delay, or a severe and enduring mental illness.

B, D: These may be options only after the OTR has an understanding of the client's occupational profile and is familiar with the client's work habits. Additionally, it is important for the client to have a realistic perspective of current skills and abilities.

Reference: Cara, E. & MacRae, A. (2005). *Psychosocial Occupational Therapy: A Clinical Practice* (2nd ed.). Thomson Delmar. Pages 597-607.

39. *Correct Answer: A*

This is the ability to recognize and react in situations as they are occurring.

Incorrect Answers:

B: This involves activating and inhibiting responses based on discrimination of stimulus information.

C: This involves memory of a past event.

D: Clients with environmental agnosia get lost in familiar places.

Reference: Zoltan, B. (2007). *Vision, Perception, and Cognition: A Manual for the Evaluation and Treatment of the Adult with Acquired Brain Injury* (4th ed.). Thorofare, NJ: SLACK, Inc. Pages 184, 195, 210, 237-239, 247.

40. *Correct Answer: C*

In the presence of complex regional pain syndrome (CRPS), vasospasm and vasodilation results in an abnormal persistence of edema. Edema control is important to include in a home program. If edema is not controlled, the protein-rich exudates causing swelling will facilitate collagen formation, resulting in joint stiffness and decrease in functional mobility/use of the hands.

Incorrect Answers:

A: Passive ROM exercises should be avoided in the presence of acute CRPS as they may aggravate the cycle of pain, swelling, and stiffness.

B: Active motion is recommended for preventing joint stiffness, maintaining differential tendon glide, and reducing edema.

D: Including instructions for energy conservation is not critical to intervention for CRPS.

Reference: Radomski, M. V. & Trombly-Latham, C. (2008). *Occupational Therapy for Physical Dysfunction* (6th ed.). Baltimore, MD: Walters Kluwer, Lippincott, Williams & Wilkins. Pages 1158-1159.

41. *Correct Answer: B*

The client's clinical symptoms are indicative of a median nerve injury. Sensory distribution for the median nerve is to the volar surface of the thumb, index, long, and radial half of the ring fingers.

Incorrect Answers:

A, C, D: These are not the typical sensory distributions for the median nerve.

Reference: Pendleton, H.M., Schultz-Krohn, W. (eds). (2006). *Pedretti's Occupational Therapy: Practice Skills for Physical Dysfunction* (6th ed.). St. Louis, MO: Elsevier Mosby. Pages 997.

42. *Correct Answer: D*

Using this approach allows the client to learn adaptive strategies, reestablish routines, and learn to function in a variety of contexts.

Incorrect Answers:

A, B, C: These approaches might be incorporated into the intervention plan for but would not be the **PRIMARY** approach for promoting progress toward the client's short-term goal.

Reference: Radomski, M. V. & Trombly-Latham, C. (2008). *Occupational Therapy for Physical Dysfunction* (6th ed.). Baltimore, MD: Walters Kluwer, Lippincott, Williams & Wilkins. Pages 55-56, 1195.

43. *Correct Answer: A*

The home program should be contextually relevant and meet the client's needs.

Incorrect Answers:

B, C: These are not effective client-centered strategies.

D: This suggests the patient will be unable to regain lost function and must rely on assistive devices.

Reference: Pendleton, H.M., Schultz-Krohn, W. (eds). (2006). *Pedretti's Occupational Therapy: Practice Skills for Physical Dysfunction* (6th ed.). St. Louis, MO: Elsevier Mosby. Pages 168, 1084.

44. *Correct Answer: C*

Clients with this muscle strength will have low endurance and will fatigue easily. This task is more demanding than the others listed because it requires the individual to locate the pants hanging in the closet and then putting the item on.

Incorrect Answers:

A, B, D: These tasks are less demanding than answer 3.

Reference: Pendleton, H.M., Schultz-Krohn, W. (eds). (2006). *Pedretti's Occupational Therapy: Practice Skills for Physical Dysfunction* (6th ed.). St. Louis, MO: Elsevier Mosby. Pages 434, 475.

Sample Items

45. *Correct Answer: C*

Providing structure and consistency is helpful for adolescents who have poor impulse control. Successful experiences help to build self-concept.

Incorrect Answers:

A, B, D: These do not adequately address impulse control or self-concept.

Reference: Bonder, B.R. (2006). *Psychopathology and Function* (3rd ed.). Thorofare, NJ: SLACK, Inc. Pages 52-54.

46. *Correct Answer: C*

Positioning and postural alignment impacts oral motor control. The OTR should evaluate the child's current seating during mealtime and recommend specific feeding positions and positioning devices.

Incorrect Answers:

A: This method is not effective to use with a child who has oral hypersensitivity.

B: Placing the neck in full forward flexion during feeding may interfere with breathing.

D: These techniques can be completed by the OTR as part of the intervention, but not by the caregiver.

Reference: Case-Smith, J. (2005). *Occupational Therapy for Children* (5th ed.). St. Louis, MO: Elsevier Mosby, Inc. Pages 502-503.

47. *Correct Answer: B*

Insidious onset of shoulder restrictions can occur due to disuse and protective posturing. It is **MOST IMPORTANT** to include ROM exercises of the unaffected joints in the intervention plan.

Incorrect Answers:

A: Positioning in a standard pouch sling should be avoided, as they promote disuse and protective posturing.

C: MCP joint blocking splints are typically not needed during the initial phase of intervention for distal radius fractures.

D: Using a dry whirlpool modality such as Fluidotherapy could potentially contaminate the external fixator pin sites.

Reference: Burke, S., Higgins, J., McClinton, M., Saunders, R. & Valdata, L. (2006). *Hand and Upper Extremity Rehabilitation: A Practical Guide* (3rd ed.). St. Louis, MO: Elsevier Churchill Livingstone. Page 492.

Radomski, M. V. & Trombly-Latham, C. (2008). *Occupational Therapy for Physical Dysfunction* (6th ed.). Baltimore, MD: Walters Kluwer, Lippincott, Williams & Wilkins. Page 1152.

48. *Correct Answer: B*

The OTR should teach the patient and caregiver to position distal end of the patient's extremity approximately 9 cm (3.5 in) above the heart. Elevation to this height allows gravity to assist with hemodynamic fluid transport.

Incorrect Answers:

A: Compression wrapping may cause adverse cyanotic changes in a hemiplegic extremity.

C: Evidence indicates that retrograde massage is not as effective as manual lymphatic drainage or elevation for managing edema.

D: PROM will help to maintain tissue length, but is not a primary means for managing edema.

Reference: Gillen, G. & Burkhardt, A. (2004). *Stroke Rehabilitation: A Function-Based Approach* (2nd ed.). St. Louis, MO: Mosby. Pages: 224-225.

Radomski, M. V. & Trombly-Latham, C. (2008). *Occupational Therapy for Physical Dysfunction* (6th ed.). Baltimore, MD: Walters Kluwer, Lippincott, Williams & Wilkins. Page 1023, 1026-1027.

49. *Correct Answer: A*

This is recommended for individuals who have limited motion for gripping small handles.

Incorrect Answers:

B: This is for clients who have lost the use of one side of the body.

C: This is for clients who have limited active motion of the hand.

D: Decreasing the weight of the utensils will not improve the client's ability to grasp them.

Reference: Radomski, M. V. & Trombly-Latham, C. (2008). *Occupational Therapy for Physical Dysfunction* (6th ed.). Baltimore, MD: Walters Kluwer, Lippincott, Williams & Wilkins. Pages 791-792, 1236-1237.

50. *Correct Answer: A*

Rhythmic initiation is a PNF technique used with individuals who have difficulty initiating motion such as is seen in Parkinson's diseases.

Incorrect Answers:

B, C, D: These are not PNF techniques.

Reference: Radomski, M. V. & Trombly-Latham, C. (2008). *Occupational Therapy for Physical Dysfunction* (6th ed.). Baltimore, MD: Walters Kluwer, Lippincott, Williams & Wilkins. Pages 704-705, 1091.

51. *Correct Answer: D*

Due to the irregular shape of the metacarpal head, the MCP joint collateral ligaments are tight when the MCP joint is in flexion. By positioning the MCP joints between 60°-70° of flexion, the MCP joint collateral ligaments will be taut and the formation of MCP flexion contractures is minimized. Positioning the IP joints in 0°-5° flexion discourages the formation of IP joint flexion contractures caused by shortening of the volar plate, collateral ligaments, and adhesions of the lateral bands.

Incorrect Answers:

A, B, C: The position of the MCP joints in these options does not maintain the optimal length of the MCP joint collateral ligaments. The position of the IP joints also promotes flexion contractures.

Reference: Pendleton, H.M., Schultz-Krohn, W. (eds). (2006). *Pedretti's Occupational Therapy: Practice Skills for Physical Dysfunction* (6th ed.). St. Louis, MO: Elsevier Mosby. Pages 1072-1075.

52. *Correct Answer: D*

A claw-hand deformity is characterized by hyperextension of the ring and small fingers (digits 4-5) and is typically caused by an ulnar nerve injury. By blocking the 4th and 5th MCP joints in flexion allows the extensor digitorum communis tendon to extend the IP joints in the absence of the ulnar innervated intrinsic muscles. The splint will enable the patient to have a more functional grasp.

Incorrect Answers:

A, B, C: These splints are not appropriate to used for a claw-hand deformity secondary to an ulnar nerve injury.

Reference: Cooper, C. (2007). *Fundamentals of Hand Therapy: Clinical Reasoning and Treatment Guidelines for Common Diagnoses of the Upper Extremity.* St. Louis, MO: Mosby. Page: 234.

Coppard, B.M. & Lohman, H. (2008). *Introduction to Splinting: A Clinical-Reasoning & Problem Solving Approach* (3rd ed.). St. Louis, MO: Mosby. Pages: 292-293.

53. *Correct Answer: D*

Using activity analysis methods it is evident that this option provides opportunity for weight bearing with the wrists in extension. This will assist in elongating the soft tissue that is inhibiting motion.

Incorrect Answers:

A, B, C: These may incorporate wrist motion, but they are not as effective for providing soft tissue stretch.

Reference: Radomski, M. V. & Trombly-Latham, C. (2008). *Occupational Therapy for Physical Dysfunction* (6th ed.). Baltimore, MD: Walters Kluwer, Lippincott, Williams & Wilkins. Pages 361-367.

Case-Smith, J. (2005). *Occupational Therapy for Children* (5th ed.). St. Louis, MO: Elsevier Mosby, Inc. Page 879-880.

54. *Correct Answer: B*

Moving from supine to sitting may result in an excessive decrease in blood pressure that reduces blood flow to the brain and results in lightheadedness.

Incorrect Answers:

A, C, D: These are not symptoms directly associated with orthostatic hypotension.

Reference: Pendleton, H.M., Schultz-Krohn, W. (eds). (2006). *Pedretti's Occupational Therapy: Practice Skills for Physical Dysfunction* (6th ed.). St. Louis, MO: Elsevier Mosby. Page 909.

55. *Correct Answer: A*

This allows optimal positioning for designated hip precautions

Incorrect Answers:

B: Clients use chair arms to push off during transfers.

C, D: These do not support positioning recommendations and precautions.

Reference: Radomski, M. V. & Trombly-Latham, C. (2008). *Occupational Therapy for Physical Dysfunction* (6th ed.). Baltimore, MD: Walters Kluwer, Lippincott, Williams & Wilkins. Pages 1120-1121.

56. *Correct Answer: B*

The client's physiologic response to activity must be monitored.

Incorrect Answers:

A, D: These may be included during Phase I but are not **ESSENTIAL** during the initial session.

C: Isometric activities are contraindicated during Phase I of cardiac rehabilitation.

Reference: Radomski, M. V. & Trombly-Latham, C. (2008). *Occupational Therapy for Physical Dysfunction* (6th ed.). Baltimore, MD: Walters Kluwer, Lippincott, Williams & Wilkins. Pages 1302-1303.

57. *Correct Answer: B*

Using a wheeled cart to transport items from one area of the kitchen to another minimizes stress on smaller finger joints.

Incorrect Answers:

A, C, D: These are not consistent with the principles of joint protection.

Reference: Radomski, M. V. & Trombly-Latham, C. (2008). *Occupational Therapy for Physical Dysfunction* (6th ed.). Baltimore, MD: Walters Kluwer, Lippincott, Williams & Wilkins. Pages 1222-1225.

58. *Correct Answer: C*

Edema reduction must be a priority of the intervention.

Incorrect Answers:

A, B, D: These interventions do not focus on reducing edema, and may be contraindicated at this stage of the treatment.

Reference: Radomski, M. V. & Trombly-Latham, C. (2008). *Occupational Therapy for Physical Dysfunction* (6th ed.). Baltimore, MD: Walters Kluwer, Lippincott, Williams & Wilkins. Pages 1153.

59. *Correct Answer: B*

Heterotopic bone formation results in loss of active ROM of the elbow. Flexion, extension and supination are typically affected.

Incorrect Answers:

A: This client is not in need of a universal cuff.

C: This is used for clients who have use of only one upper extremity.

D: These are used for clients who have no use of the upper extremities.

Reference: Pendleton, H.M., Schultz-Krohn, W. (eds). (2006). *Pedretti's Occupational Therapy: Practice Skills for Physical Dysfunction* (6th ed.). St. Louis, MO: Elsevier Mosby. Pages 168, 1084.

60. *Correct Answers: A*

Cerebellar lesions result in ataxia and dysmetria. This equipment will assist the individual to stabilize the plate and hold the cup during a meal.

Incorrect Answers:

B: A side-cutting fork and rocker knife are used for individuals who have unilateral impairment and/or those who have upper extremity weakness.

C: Lightweight equipment is typically used for individuals who have muscular weakness.

D: A universal cuff is used to substitute for a weak grasp. A mobile arm support is used in the presence of proximal arm weakness and is contraindicated for use when an individual has ataxia.

Reference: Pendleton, H.M., Schultz-Krohn, W. (eds). (2006). *Pedretti's Occupational Therapy: Practice Skills for Physical Dysfunction* (6th ed.). St. Louis, MO: Elsevier Mosby. Pages 171-172.

61. *Correct Answer: B*

This will have the **MOST** impact on kitchen safety.

Incorrect Answers:

A, C, D: These will not have a significant impact on kitchen safety.

Reference: Scheiman, M., Scheiman, M. & Whittaker, S. (2007). *Low Vision Rehabilitation: A Practical Guide for Occupational Therapists*. Thorofare, NJ: SLACK, Inc. Pages 186-187.

62. *Correct Answer: A*

The tub transfer bench provides the patient with the safest method for transferring from/to the wheelchair to the bathtub.

Incorrect Answers:

B, C, D: A shower chair or stool does not provide the patient with a safe transfer surface for transferring to either the shower or the tub.

Reference: Pendleton, H.M., Schultz-Krohn, W. (eds). (2006). *Pedretti's Occupational Therapy: Practice Skills for Physical Dysfunction* (6th ed.). St. Louis, MO: Elsevier Mosby. Page 159, 164.

63. *Correct Answer: C*

A mobile arm support attaches to a wheelchair and supports the arm at the elbow allowing the client to use residual upper extremity strength for mobility during functional activities. This device is **CONTRAINDICATED** to use if a client has a significant increase in upper extremity flexor tone or chorea movement patterns.

Incorrect Answers:

A, B, D: Clients who have these diagnoses typically experience proximal upper extremity weakness, but have sufficient ROM and adequate motor control for using a mobile arm support during ADL.

Reference: Pendleton, H.M., Schultz-Krohn, W. (eds). (2006). *Pedretti's Occupational Therapy: Practice Skills for Physical Dysfunction* (6th ed.). St. Louis, MO: Elsevier Mosby. Page 720, 887.

64. *Correct Answer: A*

After positioning the wheelchair and locking the brakes, the transfer should start with the patient moving their hips forward to the edge of the chair. Prior to standing, the patient's feet should be positioned firmly on the floor with both knees flexed to 90 degrees. This position will enable the patient to stand and pivot toward the transfer surface.

Incorrect Answers:

B: The client should not come to a standing position until the hips are moved forward to the edge of the wheelchair.

C: The OTR may ask client to rock back and forth to gain momentum for standing; but only after the hips are forward in the chair and the feet are properly positioned.

D: A client may use upper body strength to push off the wheelchair armrests, but only after the hips and feet are properly positioned.

Reference: Pendleton, H.M., Schultz-Krohn, W. (eds). (2006). *Pedretti's Occupational Therapy: Practice Skills for Physical Dysfunction* (6th ed.). St. Louis, MO: Elsevier Mosby. Page 316.

Radomski, M. V. & Trombly-Latham, C. (2008). *Occupational Therapy for Physical Dysfunction* (6th ed.). Baltimore, MD: Walters Kluwer, Lippincott, Williams & Wilkins. Page 831.

65. *Correct Answer: D*

Deep touch stimuli is typically more tolerable than light touch in the presence of tactile defensiveness.

Incorrect Answers:

A, B: Vestibular input does not necessarily improve tactile defensiveness.

C: Light touching or light stimuli is a common irritant in the presence of tactile defensiveness.

Reference: Case-Smith, J. (2005). *Occupational Therapy for Children* (5th ed.). St. Louis, MO: Elsevier Mosby, Inc. Page 378.

66. *Correct Answer: A*

To increase muscle endurance the number of repetitions must be increased while maintaining the resistance at 50% or less of maximal.

Incorrect Answers:

B: This activity will increase speed.

C, D: These activities promote increased strength.

Reference: Radomski, M. V. & Trombly-Latham, C. (2008). *Occupational Therapy for Physical Dysfunction* (6th ed.). Baltimore, MD: Walters Kluwer, Lippincott, Williams & Wilkins. Pages 361-362, 578.

67. *Correct Answer: C*

Modifying the assistive/adaptive devices, i.e., the wheelchair, by adding a solid seat to the wheelchair would aid in maintaining pelvic alignment and in providing external support. Forearm supports would provide external stability to weak upper extremity musculature. Both modifications would aid in reducing postural discomfort and muscular fatigue.

Incorrect Answers:

A: This mobility device would not allow ergonomic positioning at the client's desk.

B: A voice controlled computer system may relieve fatigue caused by typing, but does not address postural support issues caused by prolonged sitting in a sling seat wheelchair. There is no indication that the client spends a lot of time on the phone.

D: Pelvic alignment and postural support should be addressed first. There is no indication that the client needs a deltoid aid or a split design keyboard.

Reference: Pendleton, H.M., Schultz-Krohn, W. (eds). (2006). *Pedretti's Occupational Therapy: Practice Skills for Physical Dysfunction* (6th ed.). St. Louis, MO: Elsevier Mosby. Pages 210-212, 281.

68. *Correct Answer: A*

Individuals who are functioning at this cognitive level typically are able to use problem solving and inductive reasoning. Engaging this patient this type of group allows the patient to learn and try new adaptive strategies.

Incorrect Answers:

B: Contracting for safety does not teach adaptive strategies that can be used after discharge.

C: BADL is typically not affected in patients who are functioning at this level.

D: This type of structured activity is not indicated for higher-functioning patients.

Reference: Cara, E. & MacRae, A. (2005). *Psychosocial Occupational Therapy: A Clinical Practice* (2nd ed.). Thomson Delmar. Pages 249-259.

69. *Correct Answer: C*

Clients at this level typically are able to follow visual cues to perform and complete a task.

Incorrect Answers:

A: This does not promote carry-over for use when a caregiver is not present to provide the cues.

B, D: This compensatory strategy may be effective for clients who are functioning at higher cognitive levels.

Reference: Cole, M. (2005). *Group Dynamics in Occupational Therapy* (3rd ed.). Thorofare, NJ: SLACK, Inc.. Pages 183, 188-189.

70. *Correct Answer: B*

These types of contractures respond positively to serial casting and gel sheeting. The child can wear the splint intermittently during the day and all night. Functional use of the hand should be encouraged when the splint is removed.

Incorrect Answers:

A: Increasing the intensity of the exercises may be harmful to the child.

C: It is helpful to provide this information to the caregiver, but it is not the **MOST EFFECTIVE** method for dealing with the contracture.

D: This is not effective for dealing with the contracture.

Reference: Cooper, C. (2007). *Fundamentals of Hand Therapy: Clinical Reasoning and Treatment Guidelines for Common Diagnoses of the Upper Extremity.* St. Louis, MO: Mosby. Pages: 398-399.

71. *Correct Answer: A*

The ready-made cookie dough requires is most appropriate for the patient's current functional level.

Incorrect Answers:

B, C: These activities require more concentration and focus. The patient would not likely be successful in the completion of these tasks.

D: This task does not support patient's goal of completing the task independently.

Reference: Radomski, M. V. & Trombly-Latham, C. (2008). *Occupational Therapy for Physical Dysfunction* (6th ed.). Baltimore, MD: Walters Kluwer, Lippincott, Williams & Wilkins. Pages 359-368, 1048.

72. *Correct Answer: C*

The OTR should suggest strategies to increase independence without requiring adaptations that increase time required to complete task or change standard routine.

Incorrect Answers:

A, B, D: These require the client to change habits and routines without addressing the need to improve efficiency or make the task easier to complete.

Reference: Radomski, M. V. & Trombly-Latham, C. (2008). *Occupational Therapy for Physical Dysfunction* (6th ed.). Baltimore, MD: Walters Kluwer, Lippincott, Williams & Wilkins. Pages 803-804.

SECTION 5

Sample Items

73. *Correct Answer: A*

An upright orientation helps to decrease directional confusion, provides proprioceptive input for proximal control and promotes a more mature grasp pattern.

Incorrect Answers:

B: Working on a horizontal plane may be confusing for a child who has directional difficulties. This also encourages the use of a palmar grasp.

C: Cutting with adapted scissors encourages a gross opening and closing hand movement. It does not necessarily address the underlying musculoskeletal components required for a mature pencil grasp.

D: Providing hand-over-hand assistance is not an effective use of the sensorimotor approach for this student.

Reference: Case-Smith, J. (2005). *Occupational Therapy for Children* (5th ed.). St. Louis, MO: Elsevier Mosby, Inc. Pages 598-605.

74. *Correct Answer: A*

It is important to provide more external support for proper pelvic, trunk and head alignment.

Incorrect Answers:

B, C: These do not provide adequate external support for proper alignment.

D: Postural alignment is too difficult to control in this type of chair.

Reference: Case-Smith, J. (2005). *Occupational Therapy for Children* (5th ed.). St. Louis, MO: Elsevier Mosby, Inc. Pages 499-500.

75. *Correct Answer: C*

Reducing the intensity of exercises to the previous level will help to manage the client's fatigue.

Incorrect Answers:

A: Interventions should not continue if they result in fatigue.

B, D: These are not consistent with the client's current abilities.

Reference: Radomski, M. V. & Trombly-Latham, C. (2008). *Occupational Therapy for Physical Dysfunction* (6th ed.). Baltimore, MD: Walters Kluwer, Lippincott, Williams & Wilkins. Pages 1086-1090.

76. *Correct Answer: D*

This allows positioning of the trunk posterior to the pelvis and accommodates for the forces of gravity against upright positioning.

Incorrect Answers:

A, B: These are not optimal for engagement in school activities.

C: This does not address the student's intolerance for upright sitting.

Reference: Case-Smith, J. (2005). *Occupational Therapy for Children* (5th ed.). St. Louis, MO: Elsevier Mosby, Inc. Page 673.

77. *Correct Answer: A*

This change in the customary job schedule allows the client an equal employment opportunity.

Incorrect Answers:

B: The client must be able to perform essential job tasks of an accountant.

C: The employer is not obligated to provide this equipment.

D: This is not considered a reasonable accommodation.

Reference: Pendleton, H.M., Schultz-Krohn, W. (eds). (2006). *Pedretti's Occupational Therapy: Practice Skills for Physical Dysfunction* (6th ed.). St. Louis, MO: Elsevier Mosby. Pages 312-314.

78. *Correct Answer: B*

Outcomes should be measured using observable performance-based or action-oriented results.

Incorrect Answers:

A, C, D: Do not meet the criteria of measuring effectiveness of the intervention.

Reference: Fazio, L. (2008) *Developing Occupation-Centered Programming for the Community: A Workbook for Students and Professionals* (2nd Ed.). Upper Saddle River, NJ: Prentice Hall. Pages 263-281.

79. *Correct Answer: D*

Self-care tasks should be simplified and highly structured; providing simple instructions one at a time, and physical guidance during the task.

Incorrect Answers:

A, B, C: These may be appropriate as the patient's cognitive level of functioning improves.

Reference: Radomski, M. V. & Trombly-Latham, C. (2008). *Occupational Therapy for Physical Dysfunction* (6th ed.). Baltimore, MD: Walters Kluwer, Lippincott, Williams & Wilkins. Pages 1059-1060.

80. *Correct Answer: B*

Using pulleys to lift the affected arm overhead creates a risk for causing a shoulder impingement syndrome and upper extremity pain.

Incorrect Answers:

A, C, D: These are recommended for managing upper extremity spasticity.

Reference: Pendleton, H.M., Schultz-Krohn, W. (eds). (2006). *Pedretti's Occupational Therapy: Practice Skills for Physical Dysfunction* (6th ed.). St. Louis, MO: Elsevier Mosby. Pages 827-830.

81. *Correct Answer: B*

The patient should begin pursed-lipped breathing.

Incorrect Answers:

A, C: These are not pursed-lip breathing techniques.

D: Oxygen should be used during ADL if oxygen saturation falls below 88%.

Reference: Radomski, M. V. & Trombly-Latham, C. (2008). *Occupational Therapy for Physical Dysfunction* (6th ed.). Baltimore, MD: Walters Kluwer, Lippincott, Williams & Wilkins. Pages 1308-1309.

SECTION 5 Sample Items

Section Five - Sample Items   79   www.nbcot.org

82. *Correct answer: A*

The patient will benefit from learning self-management techniques. This should **INITIALLY** be done on a one-on-one basis. As progress is made, sessions can be designed to help the patient generalize techniques learned to a variety of real-life situations.

Incorrect Answers:

B, C, D: These contexts would not be **MOST** conducive for initial intervention.

Reference: Cara, E. & MacRae, A. (2005). *Psychosocial Occupational Therapy: A Clinical Practice* (2nd ed.). Thomson Delmar. Pages 210-217.

83. *Correct Answer: C*

The progression of positions should be done in incrementally small steps. In this case, the patient is sitting in a more upright position while keeping the legs in an elevated position. This allows for the blood pressure to adjust to the change.

Incorrect Answers:

A: In addition to being an inappropriate chair, the upright positioning and dependent leg position may promote orthostatic hypotension.

B, D: Positioning fully upright without elevating the legs may promote orthostatic hypotension.

Reference: Radomski, M. V. & Trombly-Latham, C. (2008). *Occupational Therapy for Physical Dysfunction* (6th ed.). Baltimore, MD: Walters Kluwer, Lippincott, Williams & Wilkins. Page 1176.

84. *Correct Answer: A*

At stage II Alzheimer's disease, the most effective recommendation to a caregiver is modifying the home environment. Using movement sensitive audio-visual assistive technology allows the client to move through the house but alerts the caregiver as to the client's activities.

Incorrect Answers:

B: The client may still wander through the home despite having this in the room.

C: This type of monitor does not have the auditory component to alert the caregiver at night.

D: This is not adequate to ensure that the client remains safely in the home.

Reference: Pendleton, H.M., Schultz-Krohn, W. (eds). (2006). *Pedretti's Occupational Therapy: Practice Skills for Physical Dysfunction* (6th ed.). St. Louis, MO: Elsevier Mosby. Page 882.

85. *Correct Answer: D*

Spontaneous use of the device is the best indicator for determining the impact of the device on an individual's functional performance.

Incorrect Answers:

A, C: The ability to use the device during OT sessions is not an indication that the resident will use the device when not in a structured intervention session.

B: The fact that a resident can verbalize what a device is used for does not mean that the resident actually uses the device during functional tasks.

Reference: Radomski, M. V. & Trombly-Latham, C. (2008). *Occupational Therapy for Physical Dysfunction*. (6th ed.). Baltimore, MD: Walters Kluwer, Lippincott, Williams & Wilkins. Pages 776-777, 807, 813.

86. *Correct Answer:* B

Goniometric measurements provide objective information to determine progress.

Incorrect Answers:

A: It is not essential to complete a sensory evaluation of the entire hand for this injury.

C, D: It is not necessary to include this information in the client contact note.

Reference: Cooper, C. (2007). *Fundamentals of Hand Therapy: Clinical Reasoning and Treatment Guidelines for Common Diagnoses of the Upper Extremity.* St. Louis, MO: Mosby. Pages: 278-282.

87. *Correct Answer:* B

This response reflects the ethical principle of nonmaleficence (Do no harm). The OTR has an obligation to do everything possible to about the benefits and risks of using the device before including it in an intervention.

Incorrect Answers:

A, C: These can be developed if the device is determined safe and appropriate for OT clinical use.

D: Reimbursements can be considered only after the device is determined safe and appropriate for OT clinical use.

Reference: Purtillo, R. (2005). *Ethical Dimensions in the Health Professions* (4th ed.). Philadelphia, PA: Elsevier Saunders. Pages 59-66, 220.

88. *Correct Answer:* C

An OT practitioner has a duty to achieve and continually maintain competency standards. Since this individual has been out of professional practice for four years, an effective learning plan should be established.

Incorrect Answers:

A: These are outdated and cannot be used to meet professional development requirements for certification renewal or licensure.

B: This individual does not meet the certification renewal or licensure requirements to practice as an OT in a volunteer capacity.

D: This individual must have proof of current professional development activities prior to submitting these applications.

Reference: McCormack, G., Jaffe, E.G. & Goodman-Lavey, M. (eds). (2003). *The Occupational Therapy Manager* (4th ed). Rockville, MD: AOTA Press. Pages 484-487.

89. *Correct Answer:* B

Since this is outside of the workplace, this has the potential to blur the boundaries of the supervisor/supervisee relationship. Thus, causing an ethical dilemma related to dual relationships.

Incorrect Answers:

A, C, D: These have clearly established boundaries that do not compromise the ethical principle of dual relationships.

Reference: Costa, D.B. (2007). *Clinical Supervision in Occupational Therapy: A Guide for Fieldwork and Practice.* Bethesda, MD: AOTA Press. Page 115-116.

90. *Correct Answer: A*

Using a question format helps to facilitate a discussion and reduces the risk of a defensive response. In this case, the student may have a valid reason for altering the test procedures, and may not be reporting standardized results.

Incorrect Answers:

B, D: This feedback invites defensive responses.

C: Beginning a feedback statement with the first person is appropriate. In this situation, the supervisor should elicit more information before providing a mandate.

Reference: Costa, D.B. (2007). Clinical Supervision in Occupational Therapy: *A Guide for Fieldwork and Practice*. Bethesda, MD: AOTA Press. Page 129.

91. *Correct Answer: B*

Gathering pertinent facts from the student opens lines of communications and helps to prevent premature judgments about the situation.

Incorrect Answers:

A, C, D: These are not appropriate for the OTR to do without initially gathering facts.

Reference: McCormack, G., Jaffe, E.G. & Goodman-Lavey, M. (eds). (2003). *The Occupational Therapy Manager* (4th ed.). Rockville, MD: AOTA Press. Pages 294-300.

92. *Correct Answer: B*

This method provides the broadest amount of information that is appropriate for this audience of the public.

Incorrect Answers:

A: This information presents a narrow focus and would be more appropriate for an audience of health care team members.

C: This does not address the diverse issues that the group as a whole may have. There are potential health information disclosure issues associated with this presentation method.

D: Generic exercise protocols may not meet individual needs and may be contraindicated for some individuals.

Reference: Fazio, L. (2008) *Developing Occupation-Centered Programming for the Community: A Workbook for Students and Professionals* (2nd Ed.). Upper Saddle River, NJ: Prentice Hall. Pages 363-364.

93. *Correct answer: B*

A letter contesting a denial of reimbursement should include evidence of functional outcomes achieved through occupational therapy intervention.

Incorrect Answers:

A,C,D: These do not address the individual's functional goals or achievements related to occupational therapy intervention.

Reference: McCormack, G., Jaffe, E., Goodman-Lavey, M. (2003). *The Occupational Therapy Manager* (4th ed.). Rockville, MD: AOTA Press. Page 409.

94. *Correct Answer: A*

The three-hour rule is a touchstone that the Centers for Medicare and Medicaid use for making an initial finding of medical necessity. The patient can continue to participate in PT for two hours per day despite being discharged from OT. It is fraudulent to continue develop a new intervention plan and/or new intervention goals if these are not medically necessary.

Incorrect Answers:

B, D: Interventions must be medically necessary and must require skilled services.

C: It is not necessary to continue OT for one hour per day just to meet the three-hour rule.

Reference: Borcherding, S.   (2005). *Documentation Manual for Writing SOAP Notes in Occupational Therapy* (2nd ed.). Thorofare, NJ: SLACK, Inc. Pages 5, 77-78.

95. *Correct Answer: A*

Level II fieldwork supervision of an OT student must be provided by an occupational therapist who has a minimum of one year of practice experience subsequent to initial certification. The supervising therapist may be engaged by the educational program or fieldwork facility.

Incorrect Answers:

C: A supervising OT must have been certified for at least one year prior to supervising a level II fieldwork student.

B, D: Although level I OT fieldwork supervision can be provided by other healthcare professionals, Level II OT fieldwork supervision must be provided by an OT who has been certified for at least one year.

Reference: ACOTE. (2007). Accreditation Standards for a Master's Level Degree Educational Program for the Occupational Therapist. *The American Journal of Occupational Therapy.* 61:6 652-661.

96. *Correct Answer: B*

Even though the co-worker is the patient's relative, there is no evidence that the patient has given signed consent to provide this relative with personal health information. The OTR should advise the co-worker of the need for patient approval.

Incorrect Answers:

A, C, D: These responses violate the patient's confidentiality rights.

Reference: McCormack, G., Jaffe, E.G. & Goodman-Lavey, M. (eds). (2003). *The Occupational Therapy Manager* (4th ed.). Rockville, MD: AOTA Press.   Page 591.

97. *Correct Answer: A*

Attestation of the NBCOT Certificant Code of Conduct is a requirement for certification renewal.

Incorrect Answers:

B: Evidence of professional development is submitted if a certificant is selected for an audit.

C, D: These are not required for NBCOT certification renewal.

Reference: NBCOT, Inc. (2008). *2008 Certification Renewal Handbook.* Gaithersburg, MD: AOTCB/NBCOT 2008 Publications. Page 16-17.

SECTION 5 Sample Items

98. *Correct Answer: A*

Initial reports should include evaluation results as they relate to a patient's overall occupational profile.

Incorrect Answers:

B, C, D: These are not essential elements of the initial evaluation report.

Reference: Borcherding, S. (2005). *Documentation Manual for Writing SOAP Notes in Occupational Therapy* (2nd ed.). Thorofare, NJ: SLACK, Inc. Pages 108-115.

99. *Correct Answer: C*

School-based OT must participation in curriculum-based activities. The physician indicates that the splints are for specifically night use, and the child is functioning at grade-level. Therefore, it is appropriate for the OTR to refer the child to a non-school-based outpatient OT clinic.

Incorrect Answers:

A: This is not appropriate practice for a school-based OT.

B: There is no need to initiate an IEP since the child is functioning at grade-level.

D: Providing this information to the parents should not be done without the appropriate OT evaluation and splint fitting.

Reference: Case-Smith, J. (2005). *Occupational Therapy for Children* (5th ed.). St. Louis, MO: Elsevier Mosby, Inc. Page 799-807.

100. *Correct Answer: D*

Sample size impacts the ability to generalize the statistical significance of a study in determining the underlying true effectiveness of an intervention.

Incorrect Answers:

A, B, C: These are not appropriate interpretations of the study's outcome.

Reference: Law, M. (2002). *Evidence-Based Rehabilitation: A Guide to Practice*. Thorofare, NJ: SLACK, Inc. Page 248-249.

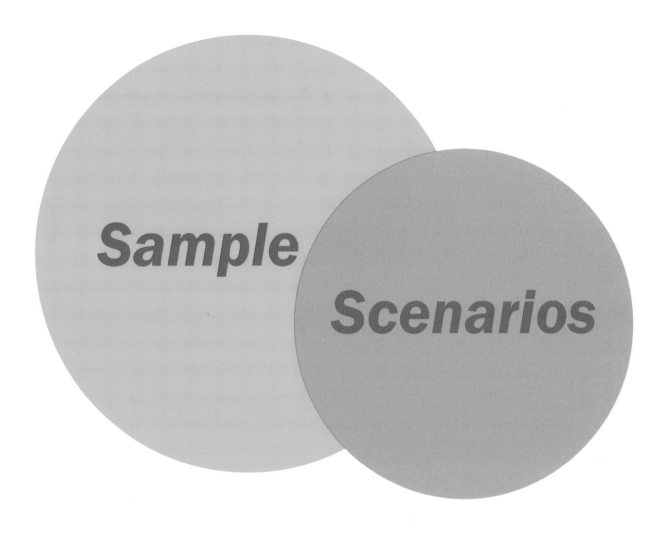

Sample Scenarios

Multiple-Choice Sample Items in Scenario Format

This section contains ten scenarios spanning a range of populations and practice settings. Each scenario has five multiple-choice items linked to an introductory passage. The domain area associated with each multiple-choice item is noted in parentheses.

As you approach each scenario, consider what you already know about the subject. Reflect on your previous experiences from fieldwork, labs, case studies, and readings. Organize the information presented in the scenario by identifying key information.

After answering each of the scenario-related multiple-choice items, grade your answers using the answer key provided. Flag any items you have scored incorrectly. Read the justification for the correct response in the answer key, and follow-up using the references provided for additional study.

An 18-month old infant with cerebral palsy is referred to outpatient OT services. A screening reveals the infant has moderate oral-sensory defensiveness and has been receiving nutritive support through a gastrostomy tube since soon after birth. The parents report the infant can only tolerate thickened pureed food due to a hyperactive gag reflex and oral motor delays. The parents' primary goal is to transition the infant to oral feeding.

1. Which activity demand is **MOST IMPORTANT** to evaluate during the initial assessment? (Domain 01)

   A. The infant's social interaction with others during play
   B. Presence of righting and equilibrium reactions when crawling
   C. Ability to manipulate developmentally appropriate toys
   D. Trunk stability when sitting in a high chair to stack blocks

2. In addition to evaluating factors that impact oral feeding, what information is **MOST IMPORTANT** to obtain when establishing a client-centered intervention plan for this infant? (Domain 02)

   A. The parents' specific childrearing styles and practices
   B. Ability of the parents to follow a designated home program
   C. Signed consent agreeing to accompany infant to all sessions
   D. Intervention outcomes from previous service providers

3. To promote goal attainment, what method or technique(s) should the OT teach the parents to do with the infant between mealtimes? (Domain 02)

   A. Provide downward pressure on the infant's tongue using a syrup-coated spoon.
   B. Rub the infant's gums with light sustained pressure using a moistened washcloth.
   C. Apply cold stimulation to the infant's tongue and soft palate using a frozen pacifier.
   D. Encourage the infant to explore the mouth using a rubber toy dipped in applesauce.

4. Which method is **BEST** for the parents to use when positioning the infant for feeding activities? (Domain 04)

   A. Holding the infant sideways in the parent's lap resting next to the parent's non-dominant arm
   B. Sitting the infant in a car seat placed on top of the dining table in directly front of the parent
   C. Having the parent kneel adjacent to the infant placed in a cradle bouncer on the floor
   D. Situating the infant in a beanbag chair placed on the couch in front of the parent

5. Which activity would be **MOST EFFECTIVE** for promoting the infant's oral motor skill development? (Domain 03)

   A. Making funny faces in the mirror
   B. Humming a simple song
   C. Giving kisses to a favorite toy
   D. Sucking a flavored ice pop

SECTION 6

Scenarios

Scenario B
A home health OTR is completing an initial evaluation with a client who has Stage 4 Parkinson's Disease. The OTR observes that the client walks with a festinating gait and uses the support of furniture and walls to maintain balance when walking from room to room. The house is cluttered, has poor lighting in hallways, and all rooms are carpeted except the bathroom. When asked about primary concerns, the client becomes tearful stating concerns about having frequent bladder accidents due to being unable to get from the living room to the bathroom in time. In addition the client reports it is difficult to change the soiled clothing.

1. Which strategy should the OTR recommend **INITIALLY** for reducing the frequency of the client's bladder accidents? (Domain 03)

    A. Placing a commode chair near to the living room
    B. Practicing pelvic floor exercises on a daily basis
    C. Reducing intake of fluids during the evening
    D. Voiding every two hours during the daytime

2. Which clothing modification should the OTR recommend for the client to successfully complete lower body dressing and undressing activities? (Domain 03)

    A. Switching belted pants for pants with an elastic waistband
    B. Replacing the pant zipper with hook and loop closure
    C. Using a button hook to fasten the pant buttons
    D. Attaching a zipper pull to a pair of front-opening pants

3. Which environmental modification should the OTR recommend **INITIALLY** in order to maximize the client's mobility within the home? (Domain 03)

    A. Replacing carpet with anti-skid strips throughout the home
    B. Clearing pathways leading to routinely used rooms in the house
    C. Installing an ECU to operate lights, television and phone systems
    D. Raising the height of bedroom and living room furniture

4. After a two-week period a re-evaluation reveals the client continues to have frequent bladder accidents. In light of the re-evaluation results, what should the OTR do **NEXT**? (Domain 02)

    A. Report the findings to the client's primary care physician
    B. Discuss additional home modifications with a family member
    C. Recommend a referral for the client to attend an adult day care facility
    D. Suggest the client use an external catheter for bladder management

5. Which administrative task **MUST** the OTR complete in order to maximize reimbursement by Medicare for services provided? (Domain 04)

    A. Write a weekly summary of observed client changes between visits.
    B. Identify new long-term goals based on remaining problems.
    C. Document each visit including client's response to services provided.
    D. Update the plan of care whenever the client's functional level changes.

An OTR working in an inpatient rehabilitation facility receives a referral for a patient who recently had a right CVA. Additionally, the patient has a history of peripheral neuropathy and glaucoma. Prior to the CVA, the patient lived in a first-floor apartment and had lately been using a standard wheelchair for community mobility due to unrelenting neuralgia. Results of the initial OT evaluation indicate the patient has moderate spasticity of the affected side, requires moderate assistance with transfers, dressing and bathing; and minimum assistance with grooming and self-feeding. The patient's spouse will provide primary caregiver responsibilities once the patient returns home. During the discharge planning meeting, the spouse asks the OTR if the patient can continue to use the standard wheelchair they already own for community outings.

1. Which of the following activities would provide the **BEST** information to evaluate the patient's visual-perceptual status? (Domain 01)

   A. Putting on a front-opening shirt
   B. Reading a newspaper article
   C. Tracking light from a penlight
   D. Ambulating across the hospital room

2. Which type of transfer surface is **BEST** to use when starting to teach the patient the sit-to-stand phase of a functional transfer? (Domain 03)

   A. Bedside chair with a cushioned seat and back
   B. Edge of a hospital bed elevated to maximal height
   C. Standard sling-seat wheelchair with swing-out leg rests
   D. Mat with high-low height adjustments

3. In preparing for discharge, which transfer technique is **BEST** to teach the spouse when assisting the patient to transition from wheelchair to bed? (Domain 03)

   A. Sliding board
   B. Stand-pivot
   C. Bent pivot
   D. Mechanical lift

4. Which of the following mobility devices should the OTR recommend for the patient's use at home? (Domain 03)

   A. Standard wheelchair with wedge cushion and pneumatic tires
   B. Power mobility scooter with a rechargeable battery pack
   C. Wheelchair with solid-seat and removable armrests and footrests
   D. Power wheelchair with folding frame and a contoured seat

5. What information should the OTR include in **INITIAL** documentation to meet Medicare reimbursement criteria? (Domain 04)

   A. Report of functional outcomes using the Minimum Data Set (MDS)
   B. Results from portions of the Outcome and Assessment Information Set (OASIS)
   C. A baseline measure of functional independence using a Patient Assessment Instrument (PAI)
   D. Expected intervention outcomes based on results from Resource Utilization Groups (RUGS)

SECTION 6

Scenarios

Scenario D

A patient who has a complete T_{12} paraplegia has recently undergone a coronary artery bypass graft surgery following a myocardial infarction. The patient is referred to occupational therapy one day after surgery. Review of the medical record indicates the patient lives alone and was independent in all IADL prior to the myocardial infarction. The patient works in a call center and enjoys competing in wheelchair races.

1. Which of the following assessments is **CONTRAINDICATED** to include in an initial evaluation with this patient? (Domain 01)

   A. Observation of BADL
   B. Manual muscle test
   C. Upper body ROM
   D. Semi structured interview

2. While observing the patient completing an upper body dressing activity while seated in a wheelchair at bedside, the OTR notes the patient's heart rate increases by 15 beats per minute above resting heart rate. Which of the following actions should the OTR take? (Domain 01)

   A. None, this is a normal physiological response to the activity.
   B. Stop the activity and assist the patient to return to bed.
   C. Seek medical assistance and monitor blood pressure.
   D. Elevate the patient's legs and observe for signs of relief.

3. Which intervention is **MOST BENEFICIAL** for the patient to learn during the initial stage of Phase I of cardiac rehabilitation? (Domain 03)

   A. Upper body graded exercise and strengthening program
   B. Methods for monitoring responses during modified transfers
   C. Energy conservation techniques to use during functional activities
   D. Purse-lipped breathing techniques for use during functional activities

4. What information is **MOST IMPORTANT** for the OTR to provide during a pre-discharge treatment team meeting? (Domain 04)

   A. Location of community-based cardiac rehabilitation programs in the area
   B. The patient's desire to resume training for an upcoming wheelchair race
   C. Modifications required at the call center prior to the patient's return to work
   D. Patient's cardiac tolerance during completion of basic self-care activities

5. The patient will require an electric hospital bed at home after discharge. What information should the OTR include in a letter of justification to a third-party payor to increase the likelihood of reimbursement? (Domain 04)

   A. Rate of recovery and progress of the patient during Phase I cardiac rehabilitation
   B. Durable medical equipment vendors that can deliver the bed to the patient's home
   C. Assistive technology the patient is currently using to complete self-care activities
   D. Purpose of the bed in enabling the patient to continue sternal precautions

An OTR working in an inpatient rehabilitation facility is evaluating a young adult who sustained an acute neurological trauma – categorized by upper motor neuron lesions – as a result of falling while playing football with friends. Screening results indicate the patient is at Level VI (confused-appropriate) on the Rancho Los Amigos Scale. The discharge plan is for the patient to return home to live with both parents who will provide caregiver assistance.

1. Which motor impairments are **TYPICALLY** associated with this type of trauma (Domain 01)

   A. Loss of voluntary muscle control with accompanying hyperreflexia
   B. Loss of voluntary muscle control with accompanying hyporeflexia
   C. Involuntary muscle control with accompanying hypereflexia
   D. Involuntary muscle control with accompanying hyporeflexia

2. What information would be **MOST IMPORTANT** to gather as part of the initial evaluation? (Domain 01)

   A. Underlying neuro-behavioral deficits that may impact long-term function
   B. Readiness and motivation to begin a functional mobility training program
   C. Patient's current visual perceptual and cognitive skills and abilities
   D. Parental report of the patient's pre-morbid cognitive skills and abilities

3. Which activity should be incorporated into the patient's **INITIAL** intervention sessions for goal progression? (Domain 02)

   A. Preparing a favorite cold snack and beverage
   B. Playing beginner-level football video games
   C. Instant-messaging friends on a computer
   D. Catching and throwing a ball at a target

4. Which type of activity would be **BEST** for the parents to use when visiting the patient at the facility during evenings and weekends? (Domain 03)

   A. Age-appropriate board games with standard rules
   B. Simple card games requiring recognition and matching
   C. Computerized games that provide immediate feedback
   D. Watching a favorite team play football on television

5. What information is **MOST IMPORTANT** for the OTR to provide to the parents during discharge planning? (Domain 02)

   A. Post-acute community rehabilitation resources
   B. Methods for monitoring caregiving fatigue
   C. Patient's maximum future vocational potential
   D. Ongoing effects of patient's injury on family dynamics

SECTION 6

Scenarios

Scenario F

An individual who has paranoid schizophrenia - and who resides at a group home - is admitted to an inpatient mental health facility after threatening another resident with a knife. The individual wants to return to the group home after discharge. Results of the initial occupational therapy evaluation indicate the individual is functioning at level 3.2 (Manual Actions) on the Allen Cognitive Scale.

1. Which functional abilities is the OTR likely to observe during an initial self-care assessment with this individual? (Domain 01)

   A. Completion of bathing and dressing tasks with verbal prompting
   B. Initiation of basic grooming tasks when visual cues are provided
   C. Scheduling of self-care tasks into a planner with moderate assistance
   D. Performing showering and grooming tasks with maximum assistance

2. Intervention planning for the individual includes attending a communication group. After the first group session the individual asks the OTR why another group member was admitted to the facility. How should the OTR respond? (Domain 03)

   A. Redirect the individual towards focusing on the content covered during the first group session.
   B. Remind the individual that information about other group members cannot be shared without their permission.
   C. Suggest the individual practices initiating conversations by asking this question to the group member during lunch.
   D. Plan to have all group members provide a brief personal history at the start of the next group session.

3. During the next communication group session the individual becomes verbally aggressive while taking part in a role-playing activity. After immediately stopping the activity, what should the OTR do **NEXT** in responding to the individual's behavior? (Domain 03)

   A. Ask the individual to identify an appropriate way to complete the task.
   B. Suggest the individual takes "time out" for the remainder of the session.
   C. Provide a written report about the incident to the individual's psychiatrist.
   D. Demonstrate correct completion of the task with accompanying feedback.

4. Re-evaluation prior to discharge indicates the individual is functioning at level 4 on the Allen Cognitive Scale (Goal-directed Actions). Which statement reflects this change and is **BEST** to include as part of the discharge summary? (Domain 04)

   A. "The individual can independently use public transportation to attend community activities."
   B. "The individual is able to complete most homemaking tasks but requires assistance with budgeting."
   C. "The individual is able to accurately compile and follow a weekly activity planner."
   D. "The individual is successful with most meal preparation tasks and could pursue a job in catering."

5. Within a month after discharge back to the group home, the individual begins talking with a disorganized speech pattern. This change is most likely a reaction to which of the following? (Domain 01)

   A. An increase in stressors within the individual's living environment
   B. Transitioning from the in-patient facility to the group home environment
   C. Side effects from psychotropic medications
   D. Cessation of taking prescribed medications

An OTR working in home health is evaluating an individual who has COPD. The individual uses a pulse oximeter for self-monitoring and supplemental oxygen through nasal canula as needed. The individual lives alone in a single-level home, has meals delivered by a community outreach service and uses public transportation for community mobility. The individual's primary concerns are progressive difficulties with self-care activities and experiencing extreme shortness of breath when taking their pet dog for a walk.

1. What should be the **PRIMARY** focus of occupational therapy intervention initially for this individual? (Domain 02)

   A. Accessing community resources to assist with pet management
   B. Safely using cleaning products during home management tasks
   C. Utilizing adaptive techniques when completing BADL tasks
   D. Using work simplification techniques to complete home chores

2. While completing a meal preparation task, the OTR notices the individual becomes short of breath and confused. What should the OTR do **FIRST** in response to this change in status? (Domain 03)

   A. Alert the individual's home health nurse.
   B. Cue the individual to modify breathing techniques.
   C. Ask the individual to rate the level of dyspnea.
   D. Check the individual's level of oxygenation.

3. Which breathing technique should the OTR instruct the individual to use to improve oxygenation? (Domain 03)

   A. Breathe in through the nose and mouth; exhale through the nose.
   B. Breathe in slowly through the nose; exhale through pursed lips.
   C. Place hands on hips and extend the spine while breathing in and out.
   D. Elevate the diaphragm when inhaling; depress when exhaling.

4. Which compensatory technique should the individual learn to use during BADL tasks? (Domain 03)

   A. Supporting elbows on the sink to brush teeth with an electric toothbrush
   B. Inhaling slowly while reaching down to the feet to put on shoes and socks
   C. Exhaling while reaching for a pair of shoes from a high shelf in a closet
   D. Using a button hook to button and unbutton front-opening shirts

5. Which technique should the individual use when preparing to take the dog for a walk? (Domain 03)

   A. Autogenic training techniques
   B. Progressive muscle relaxation
   C. Diagphragmatic breathing
   D. Visualization techniques

SECTION 6

Scenarios

Scenario H
An OTR is working with a grant-funded agency to develop a pre-vocational program for clients who have severe persistent mental illness and are participating at a day treatment center. Part of the agency's continued funding will be dependent on the success of this pre-vocational program. The OTR plans to work onsite during the program development phase and then provide intermittent consultative services to monitor program effectiveness.

1. What is the **FIRST** step of the program design process? (Domain 01)

   A. Identifying potential additional funding sources
   B. Selecting appropriate program-evaluation methods
   C. Researching existence of similar established programs
   D. Developing measurable goals based on the agency's mission

2. After developing a community and service profile, what is the **NEXT** step in conducting a needs assessment for this program? (Domain 01)

   A. Observe and monitor trends related to the clients' current time use patterns.
   B. Administer a standardized work interest checklist with a sample of clients attending the center.
   C. Interview agency representatives who are currently involved with the target population.
   D. Conduct a focus group consisting of representatives from the target population.

3. What is the **MOST EFFECTIVE** marketing tool for promoting the new program to current day center clients? (Domain 04)

   A. Display posters and brochures about the program in prominent places around the center.
   B. Include an announcement about the program during the center's weekly community meetings.
   C. Encourage clients to talk about their previous employment opportunities and experiences.
   D. Use personal sell strategies to highlight the links between program goals and client needs.

4. Three weeks after the program begins, attendance is much lower than projections. What is the **FIRST** action the OTR should take in response to these findings? (Domain 04)

   A. Write an article about the benefits of the program in the center's weekly newsletter.
   B. Talk with center staff to identify issues impacting client participation in the program.
   C. Set up a time to meet with all the clients who were initially enrolled in the program.
   D. Attend the next scheduled session to observe the staff's group facilitation skills.

5. What data would provide the **MOST** objective measure of program effectiveness? (Domain 02)

   A. Attendance levels and completion of program objectives
   B. Client satisfaction ratings obtained from end of program surveys
   C. Amount of job applications completed by the clients with minimum assistance
   D. Number of clients obtaining employment following completion of the program

Scenario I

An OTR working in an outpatient rehabilitation facility receives a referral for a 5-year-old child who one month ago sustained a non-displaced fracture of the radial head of the dominant arm following a fall during a gymnastic program. The referral states the child is experiencing increased levels of arm pain and limited functional use of the affected extremity.

During the initial evaluation, the OTR observes the child holds the affected extremity in a protected position and prefers to use the non-dominant hand for functional tasks. ROM screening indicates full active ROM of the right shoulder, -15° of elbow extension and 90° of elbow flexion. When the child attempts to make a fist, composite finger flexion of the index through small finger measures 1 inch (2.5cm) from the fingertip to distal palmar crease. Wrist extension and flexion appear to be within functional limits; but the child refuses to allow the OTR to complete goniometric measurements. The affected hand is warm to touch, with mottled skin and moderate pitting edema of the hand and fingers.

1. In addition to having decreased functional ROM secondary to the fracture, what is the child's clinical presentation **MOST** consistent with? (Domain 01)

    A. Atrophy resulting from disuse
    B. Chiralgia paresthetica
    C. Complex regional pain syndrome
    D. Interstitial compartment syndrome

2. Along with promoting engagement in purposeful activity, which intervention should the OTR plan to use to **INITIALLY** manage the child's clinical symptoms? (Domain 02)

    A. Contrast baths and progressive resistive exercise
    B. Static splinting and passive range of motion
    C. Serial casting and electrical stimulation
    D. Manual edema mobilization (MEM) and active ROM

3. What is the **MOST** accurate method for measuring change in edema in the child's hand? (Domain 01)

    A. Circumferential measurements of the hands
    B. Amount of water displacement in a volumeter
    C. Tracings of the hand positioned prone on paper
    D. Ruler measurement of composite finger flexion

4. Which of the following home activities is **BEST** for promoting a change in the child's sympathetic nervous system responses during the initial phase of intervention? (Domain 03)

    A. Drawing and erasing pictures on a dry erase board positioned on the floor
    B. Navigating through a maze of cardboard boxes while lying prone on a scooter board
    C. Throwing beanbags at a target placed at varying distances from the child
    D. Making animal shapes using graded resistance therapy putty in a variety of colors

5. Which of the following gymnastic activities – conducted in a supervised context - would support the child's goal of resuming gymnastics? (Domain 03)

    A. Walking across a 3-inch (7.6 cm) wide balance beam
    B. Tumbling forward across a mat in the gym
    C. Hanging and gently swinging from a parallel bar
    D. Swinging both legs while straddling a pommel horse

SECTION 6

Scenarios

Scenario J

An OTR receives a referral to evaluate the feeding and mobility needs of a resident in a long-term care facility who has amyotrophic lateral sclerosis (ALS). The resident currently uses both lower extremities to propel a standard manual wheelchair for short distances within the facility and requires moderate assistance of one person during functional transfers. A screening indicates that the resident's upper extremity functional strength is Poor Minus (2-/5) bilaterally. The resident reports a recent increase in incidents of coughing when eating, recurrent lower extremity muscle cramps and increased fatigue during activities. The resident's primary goal is to be able to navigate to the dining room and eat meals independently.

1. Which of the following symptoms of this disease **TYPICALLY** impacts functional performance? (Domain 01)

   A. Fasciculation and muscle atrophy
   B. Neuralgia and blurred vision
   C. Intention tremor and bradykinesia
   D. Peripheral neuropathy and hyporeflexia

2. What is the **MOST** probable cause for this resident's coughing during meal times? (Domain 01)

   A. Decreased tongue control
   B. Hyperactive gag reflex
   C. Talking to other residents
   D. Poor lip closure

3. What is the **MOST IMPORTANT** safety recommendation for the resident to follow during meal times? (Domain 03)

   A. Sit fully upright and tuck chin when swallowing.
   B. Eat warmed foods that have a pureed consistency.
   C. Eat in a quiet environment away from distractions.
   D. Use assistive devices to minimize muscle fatigue.

4. The OTR determines the resident is a candidate for a power wheelchair. What is the **MOST IMPORTANT** information to include in a letter to a third-party payor justifying funding for the power wheelchair? (Domain 04)

   A. Caregiver availability to position and supervise the resident while operating the device
   B. Resident's ability to independently participate in scheduled activities within and around the facility
   C. Motivation and willingness of the resident to learn how to use the new mobility system
   D. Benefits of the mobility device for protecting skin integrity and promoting postural alignment

5. What additional equipment should the OTR include with the order for the power wheelchair? (Domain 03)

   A. Ventilator tray
   B. Attendant controls
   C. Arm troughs
   D. Extended footplates

Scenario-Format Items

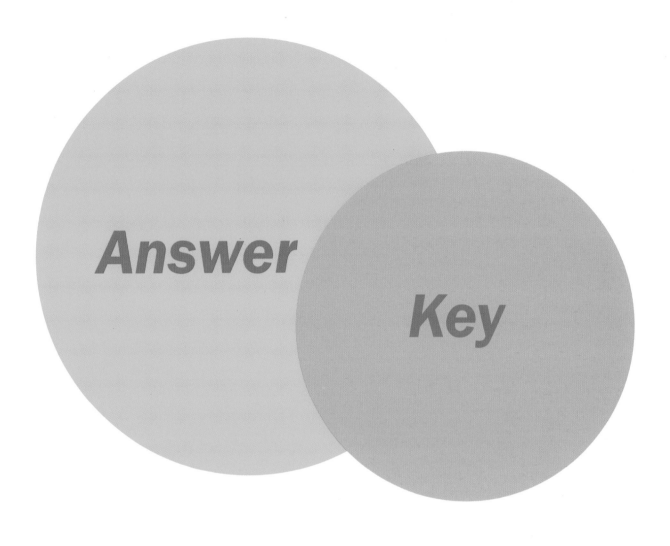

Scenarios

Scenario A

1. D
2. A
3. D
4. B
5. C

Scenario B

1. D
2. A
3. B
4. A
5. C

Scenario C

1. A
2. D
3. B
4. C
5. C

Scenario D

1. B
2. A
3. B
4. D
5. D

Scenario E

1. A
2. C
3. D
4. B
5. A

Scenario F

1. A
2. B
3. D
4. B
5. D

Scenario G

1. C
2. D
3. B
4. A
5. C

Scenario H

1. C
2. C
3. D
4. B
5. D

Scenario I

1. C
2. D
3. B
4. A
5. C

Scenario J

1. A
2. A
3. A
4. D
5. B

Scenario A

1. *Correct Answer: D*

   The infant has oral motor delays, before commencing a feeding program to assist the infant to transition to oral feeding, it is important to assess the infant's postural alignment and trunk stability.

   Reference: Case-Smith, J. (2005). *Occupational Therapy for Children* (5th ed.). St Louis, MO: Elsevier Mosby. Page 499.

2. *Correct Answer: A*

   The early intervention process recognizes that parents can be the most effective facilitator of change. It is therefore important to ascertain the specific childrearing styles and practices when collaborating with parents on designing an intervention plan for the infant.

   Reference: Case-Smith, J. (2005). *Occupational Therapy for Children* (5th ed.). St Louis, MO: Elsevier Mosby. Page 93-95.

3. *Correct Answer: D*

   Encouraging the infant to explore the mouth using a rubber toy dipped in applesauce is an effective way to desensitize and build up the infant's tolerance to oral feeding.

   Reference: Case-Smith, J. (2005). *Occupational Therapy for Children* (5th ed.). St Louis, MO: Elsevier Mosby. Page 495.

4. *Correct Answer: B*

   Placing the infant in a car seat during feeding activities is the best method to achieve postural stability and alignment for feeding.

   Reference: Case-Smith, J. (2005). *Occupational Therapy for Children* (5th ed.). St Louis, MO: Elsevier Mosby. Page 499-500.

5. *Correct Answer: C*

   Kissing is an activity that encourages active lip movements and strengthening of the oral mechanisms necessary for oral motor skill development.

   Reference: Case-Smith, J. (2005). *Occupational Therapy for Children* (5th ed.). St Louis, MO: Elsevier Mosby. Page 507.

SECTION 6

Scenarios

Scenario B

1. *Correct Answer: D*

   The client is less likely to have bladder accidents if they follow a scheduled voiding program. In addition, the client can take their time ambulating to the bathroom if their bladder is not overfull.

   Reference: Radomski, M. & Trombly Latham, C. (2008). *Occupational Therapy for Physical Dysfunction* (6th ed.). Baltimore, MD: Lippincott, Williams & Wilkins. Page 1177-1178.

2. *Correct Answer: A*

   The client has Stage 4 Parkinson's disease and is therefore likely to have decreased fine motor skills. Wearing pants with an elastic waistband will enable the client to complete lower body dressing without relying on fine motor skills.

   Reference: Pedretti, W. & Early, M. (2006). *Pedretti's Occupational Therapy: Practice Skills for Physical Dysfunction*. St Louis, MO: Mosby. Page 172

3. *Correct Answer: B*

   Due to the client's festinating gait, the client is at a greater risk for falls. Clearing pathways in the house will help to reduce the client's risk of falls.

   Reference: Radomski, M. & Trombly Latham, C. (2008). *Occupational Therapy for Physical Dysfunction* (6th ed.). Baltimore, MD: Lippincott, Williams & Wilkins. Page 1023.

4. *Correct Answer: A*

   The OTR should report the re-evaluation results to the client's primary care physician. Changes in the autonomic nervous system – including bladder function – are common with the progression of Parkinson's disease.

   Reference: Scaffa, M. (2005). *Occupational Therapy in Community-Based Practice Settings*. Philadelphia, PA: F.A. Davis. Page 201.

5. *Correct Answer: C*

   In the home health setting, a separate note must document each visit. This should include services provided and the client's response.

   Reference: Scaffa, M. (2005). *Occupational Therapy in Community-Based Practice Settings*. Philadelphia, PA: F.A. Davis. Page 218.

1. *Correct Answer: A*

   Visual perceptual skills involve the processing of visual information by the brain and motor response. Observing the patient during a functional activity requiring visual skills and motor responses – such as dressing – would provide the best information about the patient's visual-perceptual status.

   Reference: Radomski, M. & Trombly Latham, C. (2008). *Occupational Therapy for Physical Dysfunction* (6th ed.). Baltimore, MD: Lippincott, Williams & Wilkins. Page 237.

2. *Correct Answer: D*

   A high-low mat table provides a firm and stable surface from which to complete a transfer as well as enabling the OTR to control the height of the surface to promote success with this task.

   Reference: Radomski, M. & Trombly Latham, C. (2008). *Occupational Therapy for Physical Dysfunction* (6th ed.). Baltimore, MD: Lippincott, Williams & Wilkins. Page 828-831.

3. *Correct Answer: B*

   This is the best transfer to teach the patient's spouse, as it enables the spouse to safely provide assistance to the patient during the transfer if needed.

   Reference: Radomski, M. & Trombly Latham, C. (2008). *Occupational Therapy for Physical Dysfunction* (6th ed.). Baltimore, MD: Lippincott, Williams & Wilkins. Page 828-831.

4. *Correct Answer: C*

   A wheelchair with a solid-seat insert promotes postural alignment. Removable arm and footrests promotes safety during functional transfers.

   Reference: Pedretti, W. & Early, M. (2006). *Pedretti's Occupational Therapy. Practice Skills for Physical Dysfunction.* St Louis, MO: Mosby. Page 204-210.

5. *Correct Answer: C*

   Criteria for Medicare reimbursement for services provided at inpatient rehabilitation facilities is based – in part – on the measure of functional independence noted in the standard Patient Assessment Instrument (PAI).

   Reference: Braveman, B. (2006). *Leading and Managing Occupational Therapy Services: An Evidence-Based Approach.* Philadelphia, PA: FA Davis. Page 36.

SECTION 6

Scenarios

1. *Correct Answer: B*

    Individuals undergoing manual muscle testing have a tendency to hold their breath when exerting effort during the test. This causes an increase in blood pressure and slows the heart rate placing extra work on the heart. In addition, after an individual has undergone a sternotomy – a breaking of the sternum to access the heart - one-sided pulling or pushing actions with the arms must be avoided for up to six weeks following surgery.

    Reference: Radomski, M. & Trombly Latham, C. (2008). *Occupational Therapy for Physical Dysfunction* (6th ed.). Baltimore, MD: Lippincott, Williams & Wilkins. Page 1305.

2. *Correct Answer: A*

    This is a normal response to this level of activity. During the first two weeks of recovery after cardiac surgery, the heart rate should not increase more than 30 beats per minute above resting rate during exercise or activity.

    Reference: Radomski, M. & Trombly Latham, C. (2008). *Occupational Therapy for Physical Dysfunction* (6th ed.). Baltimore, MD: Lippincott, Williams & Wilkins. Page 1302.

3. *Correct Answer: B*

    Primary focus during phase I inpatient cardiac rehabilitation is to determine the patient's response to activity and prepare for discharge by practicing routine self-care activities. At this stage cardiac precautions include no lifting, pushing, or pulling with the upper extremities. Therefore it is important for the patient to be able to stay within these precautions by monitoring signs of change during modified transferred.

    Reference: Radomski, M. & Trombly Latham, C. (2008). *Occupational Therapy for Physical Dysfunction* (6th ed.). Baltimore, MD: Lippincott, Williams & Wilkins. Page 1302-1303.

4. *Correct Answer: D*

    It is the primary role of the OTR to communicate the patient's tolerated level of functioning during discharge planning. If the patient is unable to tolerate the cardiac demands of basic self-care activities, assistance of another person will be required when the patient is discharged home.

    Reference: Radomski, M. & Trombly Latham, C. (2008). *Occupational Therapy for Physical Dysfunction* (6th ed.). Baltimore, MD: Lippincott, Williams & Wilkins. Page 1302-1305.

5. *Correct Answer: D*

    A letter of justification for funding from a third-party payor for equipment should include a clear medical rationale for the requested equipment including patient's current use of the equipment and the increase in function that will be gained with the equipment use.

    Reference: Radomski, M. & Trombly Latham, C. (2008). *Occupational Therapy for Physical Dysfunction* (6th ed.). Baltimore, MD: Lippincott, Williams & Wilkins. Page 531.

Scenario E

1. *Correct Answer: A*

    A dynamic loading or impact to the head producing an acceleration, deceleration, and rotation of the brain inside the skill caused this trauma. The subsequent lesions to the upper motor neurons will result in general weakness, loss of voluntary muscle control, spasticity and hyperreflexia.

    Reference: Radomski, M. & Trombly Latham, C. (2008). *Occupational Therapy for Physical Dysfunction* (6th ed.). Baltimore, MD: Lippincott, Williams & Wilkins. Page 1044-1045.

2. *Correct Answer: C*

    The OTR should first assess the patient's vision, visual perception and cognition – to determine the extent to which the patient can scan, attend, follow and retain instructions – and use the results to guide intervention-planning decisions.

    Reference: Radomski, M. & Trombly Latham, C. (2008). *Occupational Therapy for Physical Dysfunction* (6th ed.). Baltimore, MD: Lippincott, Williams & Wilkins. Page 1057.

3. *Correct Answer: D*

    Initial intervention activities should incorporate activities to optimize motor capacities and abilities. Gross motor activities, such a ball catch/throw, minimize cognitive demands and increase focus on refinement of motor abilities. This activity also incorporates aspects of the patient's former occupation of playing football.

    Reference: Radomski, M. & Trombly Latham, C. (2008). *Occupational Therapy for Physical Dysfunction* (6th ed.). Baltimore, MD: Lippincott, Williams & Wilkins. Page 1057-1058.

4. *Correct Answer: B*

    Card games are frequently used in the early stages of rehabilitation as they can be graded to optimize cognitive capacities and abilities. Card games are typical family occupations and using them as part of therapy provides opportunities for the parents to be actively engaged in cognitive remediation activities.

    Reference: Radomski, M. & Trombly Latham, C. (2008). *Occupational Therapy for Physical Dysfunction* (6th ed.). Baltimore, MD: Lippincott, Williams & Wilkins. Page 1058.

5. *Correct Answer: A*

    Since the parents are planning to provide caregiver assistance after discharge, it is important to inform them about the full spectrum of possible TBI outcomes and availability of post-acute community rehabilitation resources.

    Reference: Radomski, M. & Trombly Latham, C. (2008). *Occupational Therapy for Physical Dysfunction* (6th ed.). Baltimore, MD: Lippincott, Williams & Wilkins. Page 1061.

SECTION 6

Scenarios

1. *Correct Answer: A*

   Individuals performing at level 3 on the Allen Cognitive Levels are able to complete basic self-care tasks, if verbal reminders are provided.

   Reference: Cole, M.B. (2005). *Group Dynamics in Occupational Therapy* (3rd ed.). Thorofare, NJ: Slack, Inc. Page 183.

2. *Correct Answer: B*

   HIPAA regulations and professional ethics require that patient information should be held in confidence and not discussed with a third party unless permission has been first granted by the individual.

   Reference: Meruani , C. & Latella, D. (2008). *Occupational Therapy Interventions, Function and Occupations*. Thorofare, NJ: Slack, Inc. Page 32.

3. *Correct Answer: D*

   Individuals performing at level 3 on the Allen Cognitive Levels require structure and assistance with problem-solving. Demonstrating the task and providing feedback would be the most appropriate method to assist the individual with attaining more appropriate communication skills.

   Reference: Cole, M.B. (2005). *Group Dynamics in Occupational Therapy* (3rd ed.). Thorofare, NJ: Slack, Inc. Page 188.

4. *Correct Answer: B*

   Individuals performing at level 4 on the Allen Cognitive Levels can complete basic ADL independently but require assistance with tasks involving planning such as money management and community transportation.

   Reference: Cole, M.B. (2005). *Group Dynamics in Occupational Therapy* (3rd ed.). Thorofare, NJ: Slack, Inc. Page 183.

5. *Correct Answer: D*

   This individual has paranoid schizophrenia. Developing a disorganized speech pattern is most likely the result of non-compliance with psychotropic medication.

   Reference: Cara, E. & MacRae, A. (2005). *Psychosocial Occupational Therapy: A Clinical Practice* (2nd ed.). Clifton Park: Thomson Delmar Learning. Page 147.

Scenario G

1. *Correct Answer: C*

   Since the individual lives alone, the primary focus of the intervention should be on maximizing independence for completing BADL safely.

   Reference: Radomski, M. & Trombly Latham, C. (2008). *Occupational Therapy for Physical Dysfunction* (6th ed.). Baltimore, MD: Lippincott, Williams & Wilkins. Page 1308.

2. *Correct Answer: D*

   Shortness of breath and confusion are signs of hypoxia. The OTR should **FIRST** take a reading of the individual's oxygen saturation using a pulse oxymeter and determine whether the individual's saturation rate is below 90% indicating oxygen is required. If the oxygen level is above 90% the individual may respond by employing pursed lip breathing while the OTR alerts the home health nurse.

   Reference: Radomski, M. & Trombly Latham, C. (2008). *Occupational Therapy for Physical Dysfunction* (6th ed.). Baltimore, MD: Lippincott, Williams & Wilkins. Page 1308.

3. *Correct Answer: B*

   Pursed lip breathing involves inhaling air slowly through the nose and exhaling through the lips as though whistling. It is the best method to use for improving oxygenation.

   Reference: Radomski, M. & Trombly Latham, C. (2008). *Occupational Therapy for Physical Dysfunction* (6th ed.). Baltimore, MD: Lippincott, Williams & Wilkins. Page 1309.

4. *Correct Answer: A*

   Individuals with COPD compensate for lack of inspiratory pressure by using their shoulder girdle muscles to expand their lungs, resulting in increased fatigue after doing unsupported upper extremity activities, such as tooth-brushing. Supporting elbows on the sink and using an electric toothbrush would assist the individual to complete this activity with less fatigue than using a manual toothbrush.

   Reference: Radomski, M. & Trombly Latham, C. (2008). *Occupational Therapy for Physical Dysfunction* (6th ed.). Baltimore, MD: Lippincott, Williams & Wilkins. Page 1309.

5. *Correct Answer: C*

   Many individuals with COPD fear extreme shortness of breath in front of others and often feel panic with breathlessness. Diaphragmatic breathing helps to slow the pace of breathing so the individual is not breathing so shallow and rapidly. Visualization may help calm the individual by mentally transporting them out of the stressful situation; however, diaphragmatic breathing is the best method to assist the individual to control the pace of breathing.

   Reference: Radomski, M. & Trombly Latham, C. (2008). *Occupational Therapy for Physical Dysfunction* (6th ed.). Baltimore, MD: Lippincott, Williams & Wilkins. Page 1310.

SECTION 6

Scenarios

Scenario H

1. *Correct Answer: C*

   Researching the existence of similar established programs will help to provide evidence that similar programming has been effective. This is an important step to complete prior to investing time and funding into conducting a full needs assessment.

   Reference: Fazio, L. (2008). *Developing occupation-centered programs for the community* (2nd ed.). Prentice Hall. Page 78.

2. *Correct Answer: C*

   It is important for the OTR to learn from agency representatives the mission and purpose of the organization along with their thoughts about current and unmet programming needs. This should be done prior to collecting data from the center's current clients.

   Reference: Fazio, L. (2008). *Developing occupation-centered programs for the community* (2nd ed.). Prentice Hall. Pages 113-115.

3. *Correct Answer: D*

   Personal selling is an effective way to describe the benefits of the new program linked to client needs. Clients with severe persistent mental illness would benefit most from this approach because it would give them an opportunity to hear first-hand why the program might be of benefit to them and provide opportunities for questions and follow-up discussion.

   Reference: Fazio, L. (2008). *Developing occupation-centered programs for the community* (2nd ed.). Prentice Hall. Pages 250-251.

4. *Correct Answer: B*

   The OTR should **FIRST** gather information from the center staff regarding issues influencing the attendance ratings of the program. This information can be then used to suggest modifications to the program as needed.

   Reference: McCormack, G., Jaffe, E., & Goodman-Lavey, M. (2003). *The Occupational Therapy Manager* (4th ed.). Rockville, MD: AOTA Press. Pages 273-274.

5. *Correct Answer: D*

   Program objectives should be performance-based and results-oriented; therefore, the best outcome data for this program is the number of clients who successfully entered employment positions after completing the program.

   Reference: Fazio, L. (2008). *Developing occupation-centered programs for the community* (2nd ed.). Prentice Hall. Pages 264-267.

Scenario I

1. *Correct Answer: C*

    Upper extremity injuries have the potential to develop complex regional pain syndrome (CRPS) – pain that is not limited to the area of initial injury. In type 1 CRPS, there is edema with abnormality of skin color or abnormal sudomotor activity. Pain that is disproportionate to the injury is a hallmark of CRPS.

    Reference: Radomski, M. & Trombly Latham, C. (2008). *Occupational Therapy for Physical Dysfunction* (6th ed.). Baltimore, MD: Lippincott, Williams & Wilkins. Page 1158.

2. *Correct Answer: D*

    Immobilization and passive range of motion are contraindicated in the treatment of CRPS. Manual Edema Mobilization (MEM) mobilizes the extracellular fluids and active range of motion moves the fluid through the lymphatic system. Repetitive isotonic contractions of the muscles in the edematous area help to drain the fluid out of the extremity. Light MEM and active movement helps to interrupt the pain cycle.

    Reference: Radomski, M. & Trombly Latham, C. (2008). *Occupational Therapy for Physical Dysfunction* (6th ed.). Baltimore, MD: Lippincott, Williams & Wilkins. Page 1159.

3. *Correct Answer: B*

    Edema is usually measured through circumferential or volumetric measurements. Volumetric measurement is more accurate, as it measures edema of the entire hand by water displacement. Circumferential measurement requires the OTR to measure at exactly the same place from test to test – and depending on where the measurement is taken – it may not account for change in total edema in the hand.

    Reference: Radomski, M. & Trombly Latham, C. (2008). *Occupational Therapy for Physical Dysfunction* (6th ed.). Baltimore, MD: Lippincott, Williams & Wilkins. Page 124.

4. *Correct Answer: A*

    A stress-loading program can be used to promote sympathetic nervous system change. Drawing and erasing pictures on a board placed on the floor is a weight bearing activity that can be graded to encourage active sustained pressure through the entire upper extremity.

    Reference: Radomski, M. & Trombly Latham, C. (2008). *Occupational Therapy for Physical Dysfunction* (6th ed.). Baltimore, MD: Lippincott, Williams & Wilkins. Page 1159.

5. *Correct Answer: C*

    Traction can be used in addition to a stress-loading program to promote sympathetic nervous system change. In a supervised context, hanging and swinging from a parallel bar will help to reduce the symptoms associated with CRPS; increase elbow motion and functional grip; and enable the child to participate in a favorite leisure skill.

    Reference: Radomski, M. & Trombly Latham, C. (2008). *Occupational Therapy for Physical Dysfunction* (6th ed.). Baltimore, MD: Lippincott, Williams & Wilkins. Page 1159.

SECTION 6

Scenarios

Scenario J

1. *Correct Answer: A*

    Fasciculations and muscle atrophy are characteristic symptoms of ALS. Sensation, vision, and bowel/bladder control are typically not affected.

    Reference: Pedretti, W. & Early, M. (2006). *Pedretti's Occupational Therapy: Practice Skills for Physical Dysfunction.* St Louis, MO: Mosby. Page 876.

2. *Correct Answer: A*

    The tongue moves the food in the mouth in preparation for swallowing. In ALS, weakness of the oral musculature can result in an inability of the person to adequately move food in the mouth in preparation for swallowing.

    Reference: Pedretti, W. & Early, M. (2006). *Pedretti's Occupational Therapy: Practice Skills for Physical Dysfunction.* St Louis, MO: Mosby. Page 876-877.

3. *Correct Answer: A*

    Head and neck positioning have a direct effect on the individual's ability to swallow and manage secretions. Incorrect positioning can lead to coughing and aspiration.

    Reference: Radomski, M. & Trombly Latham, C. (2008). *Occupational Therapy for Physical Dysfunction* (6th ed.). Baltimore, MD: Lippincott, Williams & Wilkins. Page 1331-1337.

4. *Correct Answer: D*

    Two secondary complications of ALS are pain and skin breakdown from immobility. The medical justification for ordering the power wheelchair should include: enabling the individual to be independent with basic mobility; improving respiratory function thus preventing aspiration; and maintaining skin integrity.

    Reference: Radomski, M. & Trombly Latham, C. (2008). *Occupational Therapy for Physical Dysfunction* (6th ed.). Baltimore, MD: Lippincott, Williams & Wilkins. Pages 492-493.

5. *Correct Answer: B*

    The progressive nature of ALS means compensatory techniques will need to be employed during later stages of the disease. Attendant controls will enable the resident to continue mobilization as the disease progresses.

    Reference: Pedretti, W. & Early, M. (2006). *Pedretti's Occupational Therapy: Practice Skills for Physical Dysfunction.* St Louis, MO: Mosby. Page 494-498.

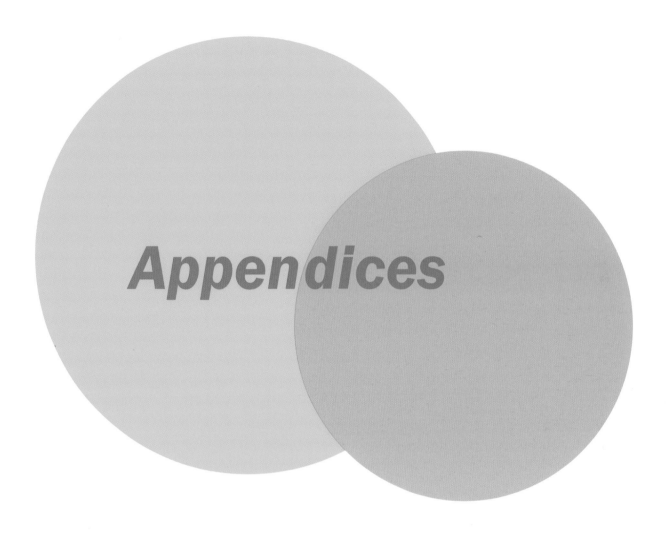

Appendices

Certification Examination Readiness Tool
for the
OCCUPATIONAL THERAPIST REGISTERED OTR®

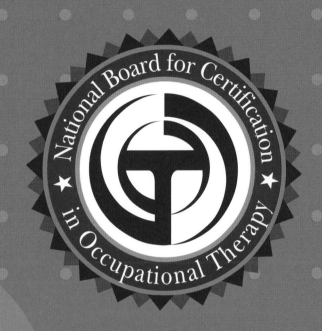

A Publication of the
National Board for Certification in Occupational Therapy, Inc.

"This tool really helped me identify my strengths and weaknesses. After using this I developed a structured study plan."

- NBCOT® Exam Candidate

"I used this tool as a part of a class assignment before the students went out on Level II fieldwork. The tool helped to formulate fieldwork goals and objectives."

- Academic Fieldwork Coordinator

"Doing this calmed my nerves... I realized that I had covered most of these skills already. It gave me confidence to continue with my exam preparation."

- NBCOT Exam Candidate

National Board for Certification in Occupational Therapy, Inc.
12 South Summit Avenue, Suite 100
Gaithersburg, MD 20877-4150
http://www.nbcot.org

𝒯*his* tool contains the validated domains, tasks, and skills resulting from the 2007 NBCOT® practice analysis study. **The tool is designed for candidates planning to take the NBCOT CERTIFIED OCCUPATIONAL THERAPIST REGISTERED OTR® examination January 2009 onwards**. It is one of several official NBCOT examination preparation tools - including study guides and online practice tests - developed to assist OTR exam candidates with their test preparation.

In line with certification industry standards, the foundation of the NBCOT certification examinations is based on a practice analysis study. NBCOT periodically conducts practice analysis studies as a basis for developing, maintaining, and defending the content validity of its certification examinations. The last practice analysis study – conducted by NBCOT in 2007 – identified the domains and tasks performed by OTR practitioners, along with the knowledge and skill required to perform them. Results from the study were used to construct the OTR examination test blueprint that will guide examination development for the NBCOT OTR certification examinations beginning January 2009.

About This Tool

This tool lists the validated domains, tasks, and skill statements used to guide examination development for the OTR certification examinations beginning January 2009.

To the right of the skill statements, there is a series of columns and corresponding checkboxes, titled:

> I have performed skill independently
> I have performed skill under supervision
> I have observed other practitioners performing skill
> I have no experience with skill

How To Use This Tool

This tool can be used in two ways to help assess readiness for the certification examination:

1. To review the validated domains, tasks and skill statements used by NBCOT item writers during the examination item development process:

    - Example of how an OTR exam item is developed:

        Domain: 04 Uphold professional standards and responsibilities to promote quality in practice

        Task: 04.05 Supervise assistants, paraprofessionals, students, and volunteers in accordance with professional guidelines and applicable regulations in order to support the delivery of appropriate occupational therapy services.

        Skill: a)   Delegating tasks and responsibilities to supervisees as appropriate

        Exam Item: An OTR is supervising an entry-level COTA who has achieved service competency. Which of the following clinical tasks can the COTA perform under close supervision from the OTR?

        A. Select appropriate assessments for new patient referrals.
        B. Administer specific standardized assessments.*
        C. Discontinue services based on patient outcomes.
        D. Establish the duration and frequency of patient treatment

        *correct answer

Appendices

A

2. As a self-evaluation tool, the user may choose to indicate their level of experience for each skill by marking the corresponding checkbox.

Example of self-evaluation:

Skill	Performed independently	Under supervision	Observed others	No experience
04.04 Articulate how occupational therapy contributes to beneficial outcomes for clients and relevant others based on evidence in order to promote quality care.				
a. Clarifying the role, responsibilities, and scope of practice for OT practitioners	√			
b. Developing and disseminating information about OT services			√	

Disclaimer: Using this tool cannot guarantee your success on the NBCOT® certification examination. However, candidates may consider using the tool to guide their test preparation strategies or as a basis for discussion with their program director or fieldwork educator.

Skill	Performed independently	Under supervision	Observed others	No experience
01.01 Evaluate the client on an ongoing basis using appropriate tools, procedures, and protocols in order to determine factors that impact participation in occupation.				
a. Conducting oneself in a therapeutic manner to gather essential data				
b. Identifying client needs, problems, concerns, and priorities about occupations and daily life activity performance				
c. Identifying factors that support or hinder occupational performance				
d. Gathering client history as a reference to activities and engagement in occupations				
e. Selecting, administering, and scoring appropriate screening and/or assessment instruments				
f. Modifying assessments based on client needs and/or performance				
g. Recognizing and responding to unexpected client responses				
01.02 Identify environments and contexts using appropriate theoretical approaches or models of practice in order to determine facilitators and/or barriers that impact the client's participation in occupation.				
a. Using appropriate theoretical approaches or models of practice to identify environmental and contextual factors that support or hinder occupational performance				
b. Obtaining information in accordance with regulatory, funding requirements, and levels of service provision				

Skill	Performed independently	Under supervision	Observed others	No experience
02.01 Interpret the evaluation results and available evidence regarding the impact of current condition(s) and context(s) on the client's occupational performance in order to determine the need for occupational therapy services and support intervention planning (includes interpreting and measuring client outcomes based on reevaluation results).				
a. Using evidence to support clinical decision-making				
b. Interpreting quantitative and qualitative evaluation data accurately				
c. Using critical reasoning to formulate conclusions about factors that impact occupational performance				
d. Identifying activities to enhance the client's occupational performance				

Appendices A

Skill	Performed independently	Under supervision	Observed others	No experience
02.02 Collaborate with the client and relevant others using a team approach in order to prioritize client-centered goals throughout the continuum of care, guided by evidence and the principles of best practice.				
a. Identifying a variety of team roles and responsibilities				
b. Communicating with the client and team members about client goals and outcomes				
c. Facilitating client participation to prioritize needs and identify goals				
d. Developing measurable and culturally relevant goals				
e. Using appropriate criteria to formulate a discharge plan				
f. Formulating and implementing a discharge plan				
g. Communicating the recommended discharge plan to the client and relevant others				
h. Identifying appropriate transitional services				
02.03 Develop an occupation-based intervention plan by selecting intervention strategies and approaches consistent with prioritized needs and best practice in order to facilitate client outcomes.				
a. Selecting the appropriate frame of reference				
b. Using occupation in a therapeutic manner to promote function based on client roles, habits and routines and current abilities				
c. Analyzing activities for the selection of occupation-based interventions consistent with client roles, habits, routines, and current abilities				
d. Selecting the intervention environment to support participation in occupation				
e. Identifying appropriate interventions using best practice as a guide				
f. Implementing methods and techniques to promote carry-over of interventions within the transitional environment, home, work, school and/or community				
g. Determining frequency and duration of intervention based on expected outcomes				

Skill	Performed independently	Under supervision	Observed others	No experience
02.04 Determine the need for referral to other professionals or services using evaluation results in order to facilitate comprehensive, quality care.				
a. Identifying parameters of other service delivery models (e.g., criteria, least restrictive environment, acuity)				
b. Identifying the roles of other service providers to determine appropriate referral and community resources				
c. Locating and communicating with other service providers and community organizations				

03 SELECT AND IMPLEMENT EVIDENCE-BASED INTERVENTIONS TO SUPPORT PARTICIPATION IN AREAS OF OCCUPATION (e.g., ADL, education, work, play, leisure, social participation) THROUGHOUT THE CONTINUUM OF CARE

Skill	Performed independently	Under supervision	Observed others	No experience
03.01 Use critical reasoning to select and implement interventions and approaches consistent with general medical, neurological, and musculoskeletal conditions and client needs in order to achieve functional outcomes within areas of occupation.				
a. Conducting oneself in a therapeutic manner to facilitate change based on a client's general medical, neurological, and/or musculoskeletal condition				
b. Selecting and implementing compensatory, remedial, biomechanical and/or preventive interventions as related to general medical, neurological, and/or musculoskeletal conditions				
c. Facilitating individual and group occupation-based activities consistent with a client's general medical, neurological, and/or musculoskeletal condition and current abilities				
d. Using facilitation and handling principles and techniques consistent with general medical, neurological, and/or musculoskeletal condition				
e. Incorporating physical agent modalities in the intervention as an adjunct to participation in functional activities				
f. Selecting, designing, fabricating and/or modifying splints and/or modifying splints and orthotic devices consistent with general medical, neurological, and/or musculoskeletal conditions and client needs				
g. Selecting, designing, fabricating and/or modifying adaptive equipment or assistive devices consistent with general medical, neurological, and/or musculoskeletal conditions and client needs				
h. Using evidence-based interventions to promote chewing and swallowing specific to general medical conditions				
i. Teaching positioning and physical transfer techniques relative to activity demands, and the client's current abilities. Using neurobehavioral approaches and techniques to promote skill development.				

Appendices

A

Skill	Performed independently	Under supervision	Observed others	No experience
03.02 **Use critical reasoning to select and implement interventions and approaches consistent with developmental level, pediatric conditions, and/or congenital anomalies and client needs in order to achieve functional outcomes within areas of occupation.**				
a. Using occupation in a therapeutic manner to promote developmental skills and abilities				
b. Conducting oneself in a therapeutic manner to facilitate change consistent with developmental needs				
c. Selecting and implementing interventions consistent with developmental level, pediatric conditions and/or congenital conditions				
d. Using developmentally-based methods and techniques to facilitate group activities				
e. Using facilitation and handling techniques during interventions consistent with developmental level, pediatric conditions, and/or congenital anomalies				
f. Using sensory integrative interventions and sensory modulation techniques during intervention				
g. Selecting, designing, fabricating and/or modifying splints and orthotic devices consistent with developmental level, pediatric conditions, and/or congenital anomalies and client needs				
h. Selecting, designing, fabricating and/or modifying adaptive equipment or assistive devices consistent with developmental level, pediatric conditions, and/or congenital anomalies and client needs				
i. Using evidence-based interventions for facilitating chewing and swallowing specific to developmental level, pediatric conditions, and/or congenital anomalies				
j. Teaching positioning and physical transfer techniques consistent with developmental level and activity demands				
k. Using neurobehavioral approaches and techniques for skill acquisition consistent with developmental level, pediatric conditions, and/or congenital anomalies				
l. Using prevocational and vocational explorations processes and procedures				
03.03 **Use critical reasoning to select and implement interventions and approaches consistent with psychosocial and cognitive abilities, and client needs in order to facilitate outcomes within areas of occupation.**				
a. Using occupation in a therapeutic manner appropriate to psychosocial and/or cognitive abilities, client roles, habits and routines				
b. Selecting and implementing therapeutic interventions appropriate to psychosocial or cognitive abilities, client roles, habits and routines				
c. Conducting oneself in a therapeutic manner to facilitate change based on psychosocial and/or cognitive abilities				

Skill	Performed independently	Under supervision	Observed others	No experience
d. Using compensatory, remedial, and/or preventive strategies consistent with psychosocial and/or cognitive abilities, client roles, habits and routines				
e. Selecting, designing, fabricating and/or modifying adaptive equipment or assistive devices based on psychosocial and/or cognitive abilities				
f. Designing and facilitating group activities consistent with psychosocial and/or cognitive models of practice				
g. Responding in a therapeutic manner to the needs of a client or caregiver during psychosocial interventions				
03.04 Maximize accessibility to and mobility within a client's contexts by identifying and recommending environmental modifications in order to optimize occupational performance and/or enhance quality of life.				
a. Analyzing environment for accessibility and risk				
b. Assessing mobility, seating, assistive technology, and durable medical equipment needs				
c. Selecting seating and mobility systems, durable medical equipment, environmental modifications, and/or assistive technology				
d. Making environmental modifications to support participation in occupation				
e. Collaborating with the client and/or relevant others regarding the need for environmental modifications, community mobility, mobility device, and/or durable medical equipment needs and options				
f. Communicating with the client and relevant others (e.g., family, team members, vendors, payors) to acquire devices				
g. Evaluating the effectiveness of modifications and/or devices within areas of occupation				
h. Educating and training the client and relevant others about the safe and effective use of environmental modifications, seating and mobility devices, durable medical equipment, and assistive technology				
i. Identifying and managing adverse reactions to environmental modifications				
03.05 Modify interventions based on the client's needs and responses in order to promote occupational performance.				
a. Identifying the need adjust intervention techniques, adapt the intervention environment, and/or grade the intervention activity				
b. Adjusting the intervention method or technique in response to variances from anticipated outcomes				
c. Adapting the environment to support participation during the intervention				
d. Grading the intervention activity based on expected progress and/or unexpected physical responses				
e. Responding appropriately to unexpected occurrences during intervention				

Skill	Performed independently	Under supervision	Observed others	No experience
03.06 Apply the principles of health promotion, wellness, prevention and/or educational programming based on client and community needs in order to provide information or serve as a resource consultant for occupation based program activities.				
a. Identifying service needs for various populations				
b. Advocating for services and resources for various populations				
c. Designing and implementing programs for at-risk populations				
d. Designing and conducting individual and group health promotion and wellness activities				
e. Collaborating with community-based agencies (e.g., senior centers, homeless shelter, service providers, funding agencies)				

04 UPHOLD PROFESSIONAL STANDARDS AND RESPONSIBILITIES TO PROMOTE QUALITY IN PRACTICE

Skill	Performed independently	Under supervision	Observed others	No experience
04.01 Maintain ongoing competence by participating in professional development activities and appraising evidence-based literature using critical reasoning skills in order to provide effective services and promote quality care.				
a. Identifying appropriate professional development activities				
b. Adapting to changes in practice due to advances in the OT body of knowledge				
c. Interpreting results and conclusions				
d. Applying evidence-based knowledge to practice				
e. Creating a professional development plan				
04.02 Uphold professional standards by participating in continuous quality improvement activities and complying with safety regulations, laws, ethical codes, facility policies and procedures, and guidelines governing OT practice in order to protect the public interest.				
a. Complying with federal, state, and other types of regulatory laws and rules				
b. Identifying policies and procedures that are specific to agencies				
c. Implementing safety and risk management techniques during intervention				
d. Incorporating federally mandated guidelines into intervention plans				
e. Designing and implementing safeguards in an environment to promote safety				

Skill	Performed independently	Under supervision	Observed others	No experience
f. Collecting, interpreting, and analyzing outcomes data				
g. Developing an improvement plan				
h. Advocating changes that improve quality of care				
i. Organizing time and services				
04.03 Document occupational therapy services and outcomes using established guidelines in order to verify accountability and to meet the requirements of practice settings, accrediting bodies, regulatory agencies and/or funding sources.				
a. Organizing documentation accurately and in accordance with practice setting, regulatory agencies or funding sources				
b. Differentiating among financial systems for reimbursement purposes				
c. Communicating effectively through documentation				
d. Adhering to applicable regulations and guidelines related to documentation				
04.04 Articulate how occupational therapy contributes to beneficial outcomes for clients and relevant others based on evidence in order to promote quality care.				
a. Clarifying the role, responsibilities, and scope of practice for OT practitioners				
b. Developing and disseminating information about OT services				
04.05 Supervise assistants, paraprofessionals, students, and volunteers in accordance with professional guidelines and applicable regulations in order to support the delivery of appropriate occupational therapy services.				
a. Delegating tasks and responsibilities to supervisees as appropriate				
b. Communicating and collaborating effectively with supervisees				
c. Assessing the competence of supervisees				
d. Incorporating competency-based learning activities				
e. Developing remedial plans				

Appendices

A

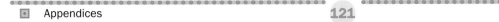

National Board for Certification in Occupational Therapy, Inc.
12 South Summit Avenue, Suite 100
Gaithersburg, MD 20877-4150
P: 301.990.7979   F: 301-869.8492
www.nbcot.org

ACOTE. (2007). Accreditation Standards for a Master's Level Degree Educational Program for the Occupational Therapist. *The American Journal of Occupational Therapy.*

Asher, I.E. (2007). *Occupational Therapy Assessment Tool: An Annotated Index (3rd ed.).* Bethesda, MD: AOTA Press.

*Barnhart, P.A. (1997). *The Guide to National Professional Certification Programs (2nd ed.).* Amherst, MA: HRD Press.

*Brookfield, S. (1987). *Developing Critical Thinkers.* San Francisco, CA: Jossey-Bass, Inc.

Borcherding, S. & Morreale, M. (2005). *The OTA's Guide to Writing SOAP Notes (2nd ed.).* Thorofare, NJ: SLACK, Inc.

Braveman, B. (2006). *Leading and Managing Occupational Therapy Services: An Evidence-Based Approach.* Philadelphia, PA: F.A. Davis.

Bonder, B.R. (2006). *Psychopathology and Function (3rd ed.).* Thorofare, NJ: SLACK, Inc.

Bruce, M. & Borg, B. (2002). *Psychosocial Frames of Reference: Core for Occupation-based Practice (3rd ed.).* Thorofare, NJ: SLACK, Inc.

Burke, S., Higgins, J., McClinton, M., Saunders, R., & Valdata, L. (2006). *Hand and Upper Extremity Rehabilitation: A Practical Guide (3rd ed.).* St. Louis, MO: Elsevier, Churchill, Livingstone.

Cara, E, & MacRae, A. (2005). *Psychosocial Occupational Therapy: A Clinical Practice (2nd ed.).* NY: Thomson Delmar.

Case-Smith, J. (2005). *Occupational Therapy for Children (5th ed.).* St. Louis, MO: Elsevier Mosby.

Cole, M.B. (2005). *Group Dynamics in Occupational Therapy: The Theoretical Basis and Practice Application of Group Intervention (3rd ed.).* Thorofare, NJ: SLACK, Inc.

Cooper, C. (2007). *Fundamentals of Hand Therapy: Clinical Reasoning and Treatment Guidelines for Common Diagnoses of the Upper Extremity.* St. Louis, MO: Elsevier Mosby.

Coppard, B.M. & Lohman, H. (2008). *Introduction to Splinting: A Clinical-Reasoning & Problem Solving Approach (3rd ed.).* St. Louis, MO: Elsevier Mosby.

Costa, D.B. (2007). *Clinical Supervision in Occupational Therapy: A Guide for Fieldwork and Practice.* Bethesda, MD: AOTA Press.

*Covey, S.R. (1989). *The 7 Habits of Highly Effective People.* New York: Simon & Schuster.

Davis, C.M. (2006). *Patient Practitioner Interaction: An Experiential Manual for Developing the Art of Health Care (4th ed.).* Thorofare, NJ: SLACK, Inc.

Fazio, L. (2008). *Developing Occupation-Centered Programming for the Community: A Workbook for Students and Professionals (2nd ed.).* Upper Saddle River, NJ: Prentice Hall.

Gentile, M. (2005). *Functional Visual Behavior in Children: A Guide to Evaluation and Treatment Options (3rd ed.)*. Bethesda, MD: AOTA Press.

Gillen, G., & Burkhardt, A. (2004). *Stroke Rehabilitation: A Function-Based Approach (2nd ed.)*. St. Louis, MO: Mosby.

Law, M. (2002). *Evidence-Based Rehabilitation: A Guide to Practice*. Thorofare, NJ: SLACK, Inc.

Mandel, Jackson, Zemke, Nelson & Clark. (1999). *Implementing the Well Elderly Program*. MD: AOTA Press.

*McClain, N., Richardson, B., & Wyatt, J. (2004, May-June). A profile of certification for pediatric nurses. *Pediatric Nursing*, 207-211.

McCormack, G., Jaffe, E.G. & Goodman-Lavey, M. (eds). (2003) *The Occupational Therapy Manager (4th ed.)*. Rockville, MD: AOTA Press.

Meriano, C. & Latella, D. (2008). *Occupational Therapy Interventions, Function and Occupations*. Thorofare, NJ: Slack, Inc.

*Microsoft (2003). Microsoft certifications benefits of certification. Retrieved from *www.microsoft.com/traincert*.

NBCOT, Inc. (2008). *2008 Certification Renewal Handbook*. Gaithersburg, MD: AOTCB/NBCOT 2008 Publications.

Pedretti, W. & Early, M. (2006). *Pedretti's Occupational Therapy: Practice Skills for Physical Dysfunction (6th ed.)*. St. Louis, MO: Elsevier Mosby.

Purtillo, R. (2005). *Ethical Dimensions in the Health Professions (4th ed.)*. Philadelphia, PA: Elsevier Saunders.

Radomski, M.V. & Trombly-Latham, C. (2008). *Occupational Therapy for Physical Dysfunction (6th ed.)*. Baltimore, MD: Lippincott, Williams and Wilkins.

Sames, K. (2005). *Documenting Occupational Therapy Practice*. New Jersey: Pearson Prentice Hall.

Scaffa, M. (2005). *Occupational Therapy in Community-based Practice Settings*. Philadelphia, PA: F.A. Davis.

Scheiman, M., Scheiman, M. & Whittaker, S. (2007). *Low Vision Rehabilitation: A Practical Guide for Occupational Therapists*. Thorofare, NJ: SLACK, Inc.

Watson, D.E. & Wilson, S.A. (2003). *Task Analysis: An Individual and Population Approach (2nd ed.)*. Bethesda, MD: AOTA Press.

Zoltan, B. (2007). *Vision, Perception, and Cognition: A Manual for the Evaluation and Treatment of the Adult with Acquired Brain Injury (4th ed.)*. Thorofare, NJ: SLACK, Inc.

---

*   *References cited during introductory chapter of this study guide. These references should not be viewed as examination item references.*

The following is a list of abbreviations (acronyms) that are to be used in examination items:

ADA	=	The Americans with Disabilities Act
ADL	=	Activities of Daily Living (not ADLs or ADL's)
AIDS	=	Acquired Immune Deficiency Syndrome
BADL	=	Basic Activities of Daily Living
COPD	=	Chronic Obstructive Pulmonary Disease
COTA	=	CERTIFIED OCCUPATIONAL THERAPY ASSISTANT COTA®
CPR	=	Cardiopulmonary Resuscitation
CVA	=	Cerebrovascular Accident
DIP	=	Distal Interphalangeal*
DSM IV	=	Diagnostic and Statistical Manual of Mental Disorders - 4th Ed.
HIPAA	=	Health Information Portability and Accountability Act
HIV	=	Human Immunodeficiency Virus
IADL	=	Instrumental Activities of Daily Living
IEP	=	Individual Education Program
MCP	=	Metacarpophalangeal
MP	=	Metacarpophalangeal
NDT	=	Neuro-Developmental Treatment
OTR	=	OCCUPATIONAL THERAPIST REGISTERED OTR®
PADL	=	Personal Activities of Daily Living
PIP	=	Proximal Interphalangeal*
ROM	=	Range of Motion
SCI	=	Spinal cord injury
SOAP	=	Subjective, Objective, Assessment, Plan Components of the Problem-Oriented Medical Record
TBI	=	Traumatic Brain Injury
TTY/TDD	=	Teletypewriter/telecommunication device for the deaf

*Must be followed by the word "joint"

Diagnoses/Conditions

ADHD
Adjustment disorders
Alcohol/substance abuse
Amyotrophic Lateral Sclerosis
Alzheimer's Disease
Amputation/Prostheses
Anxiety disorders
Aphasia
Apraxia
Arthritis/Collagen Injury
Ataxia/Incoordination
Autism
Autonomic Dysreflexia
Back Pain
Balance
Bipolar disorders
Blood pressure/hypertension
Body scheme/apraxia/neglect
Burns
Cardiopulmonary disease
COPD
Ischemia
Respiratory
Carpal tunnel
Cognitive dysfunction
Cerebral Palsy
Complex Regional Pain Syndrome
Cumulative trauma disorders
    DeQuervain's Disease
    Carpal Tunnel Syndrome
    Lateral Epicondylitis
    Cubital Tunnel Syndrome
CVA/Hemiplegia
Death/Dying/Hospice
Decubitis Ulcers
Deep Vein Thrombosis
Dementia/Alzheimer's/Memory
Depression
Desensitization

Developmental Disorders
    Autism
    Asperger's
    Developmental Delay
    Down Syndrome
Diabetes
Distractibility/Concentration
Domestic violence/Abuse—Child/Spousal/
    Elder
Dysphagia/Swallow
Dyspraxia
Eating disorders
Edema
Encephalopathy
Falls
Fetal Alcohol Syndrome
Fibromyalgia
Figure ground
Flexibility/flexion
Fractures
Grasp/grip
Guillain Barré
Hand Injury
Hemiplegia/hemiparesis
Heterotropic Ossification
Hip/Knee/Joint replacement
HIV/AIDS
Hypertonia/spasticity
Hypotonicity/flaccidity
Joints/MCP/PIP
Learning disabilities
Muscular Dystrophy
Medications/Side Effects
Motor skills/planning/control
Motor skills/planning/control
Mental Retardation
Multiple Sclerosis
Muscle tone
Neurodevelopmental Treatment (NDT)

Nerve injuries/Peripheral Neuropathy
Normal Child Development
Oral/Tongue
OCD
Osteoporosis
Pain
Paralysis
Parkinson's/tremors
Perception
Perserveration
Personality disorder
Pervasive Developmental Disorder
Positioning/Trunk control
Post-polio Syndrome
Post Traumatic Stress Disorder
Postural Hypotension
Reading disorders
Reflexes
ATNR
STNR
Labyrinthine
Head Righting
ROM/PROM
Schizophrenia
SCI
      Paraplegia
      Tetraplegia
      Quadriplegia
Sensation
Sensory Integrative Disorders
Sequencing
Scar Remodeling—
Hypertrophic scar
Spasticity
Spina Bifida
Suicidal Ideation
Tactile defensiveness
Tardive Dyskinesia
TBI
Tenosynovitis/deQuervain's
Tonic bite
Vision impairments
      Low Vision
Macular degeneration
Homonymous hemianopsia
Work-related injuries

Interventions/Treatments/Equipment

Activities of Daily Living (ADL)
Age-appropriate/Graded activity
Augmentative Communication
Assessment tools
Assistive/Adaptive Environment
Assistive Devices
Adaptiveutensils Assistive technology
Behavior Modification
Biomechanical
Body Mechanics
Chaining
Forward chaining
Backward chaining
Client-Centered Approaches
Cognitive–Perceptual Retraining
Community Integration
Community Referrals
Compensatory Techniques
Coping Strategies
Desensitization
Discharge Planning
Energy Conservation
Endurance/strength/exercise
Environmental Modification
Ergonomics
Goal-Setting
Graded activities
Group dynamics
Home program education
Joint Protection
Lifestyle redesign
Muscle testing
Patient Education
Positioning
Pressure garments
Purposeful Activity
Range of Motion Exercises
Role play
Safety
Universal Precautions
Sanitation
Sensory Reeducation
Splint Fabrication/Modification
Strengthening Exercises

Appendices

D

Transfer Training/Education
Wheelchair Assessment/Modification
Wheelchair/Functional Mobility
Work Hardening/Functional Capacity
Work Simplification

Service Components

Communication skills
Confidentiality
Conflict of Interest
Cultural Sensitivity/Diversity
        Culturally responsive care
COTA/OTR roles & responsibilities
CQI/Performance improvement
Discharge Planning/Documentation Methods
Documentation Method/Responsibilities
Evaluation/Reevaluation
Frames of Reference / Models of Practice
Informed consent
Insurance authorization/reimbursement
Interviewing skills/methods
Multidisciplinary Team Process
        Listening
Negotiating
Conflict resolution
        Roles & responsibilities
Professional Liability
Program evaluation
Promoting the Profession
Refusal of service
Research methods
Reliability
Validity
Research design
Resource Management
        Time
Equipment
Supplies
Screening
Service Collaboration
Service Competencies
Strategic planning/goals

Settings/Situations

Acute Care Hospital
Adult Daycare Center
ADA
Architectural/Environmental barriers
Assisted Living Facilities
Automobile
Bathing/Bathroom
Classroom
Clinic
Cooking
Community-based
Consultant
Daycare Facility
Dressing
Eating/Dining
Grooming/hygiene
Groups—Inpatient/Outpatient
Group Home
Home-based
IDEA
Independence
Inpatient Rehab Facility
Interests
Job elements
Leisure
Long-term care facility
Occupation
Playground
Play/leisure activities
Prison/Confinement Facility
School-based
Skilled Nursing Facility
Toileting
Treatments—New/Unfamiliar
Volunteers
Wellness programs
Workplace
Writing/prewriting

DOMAIN:

01 GATHER INFORMATION REGARDING FACTORS THAT INFLUENCE OCCUPATIONAL PERFORMANCE

TASK:

01.01 *Evaluate the client on an ongoing basis using appropriate tools, procedures, and protocols in order to determine factors that impact participation in occupation.*

Knowledge of:

01.01.01	Information gathering processes and procedures (e.g., observation, interview, client records)
01.01.02	Administration and scoring of standardized/non-standardized screening and assessment instruments
01.01.03	Normal development and function across the lifespan
01.01.04	Expected patterns/progressions associated with conditions that limit occupational performance
01.01.05	Client contexts (cultural, physical, social, personal, spiritual, temporal, and virtual)
01.01.06	Activity demands
01.01.07	Methods for responding appropriately to unexpected occurrences during the data gathering process

TASK:

01.02 *Identify environments and contexts using appropriate theoretical approaches or models of practice in order to determine facilitators and/or barriers that impact the client's participation in occupation.*

Knowledge of:

01.02.01	Theoretical approaches and models of practice
01.02.02	Facilitators and/or barriers to participation in occupation
01.02.03	Site assessment processes and procedures (e.g., work, home, school, community)
01.02.04	Impact of environments on development and occupational performance
01.02.05	Resources and support systems currently available to the client

Appendices

E

DOMAIN:

02 FORMULATE CONCLUSIONS REGARDING THE CLIENT'S NEEDS AND PRIORITIES TO DEVELOP A CLIENT-CENTERED INTERVENTION PLAN

TASK:

02.01 *Interpret the evaluation results and available evidence regarding the impact of current condition(s) and context(s) on the client's occupational performance in order to determine the need for occupational therapy services and support intervention planning (includes interpreting and measuring client outcomes based on reevaluation results).*

Knowledge of:

02.01.01	Clinical decision-making and critical reasoning
02.01.02	Tools and techniques for interpreting data
02.01.03	Internal and external influences on occupational performance (e.g., disability, environment, context, medication)
02.01.04	Activities that can enhance occupational performance

TASK:

02.02 *Collaborate with the client and relevant others using a team approach in order to prioritize client-centered goals throughout the continuum of care, guided by evidence and the principles of best practice.*

Knowledge of:

02.02.01	Team roles, responsibilities and care coordination
02.02.02	Collaborative client-centered strategies
02.02.03	Goal formulation based on expected outcomes of intervention
02.02.04	Discharge planning procedures
02.02.05	Transitional services

TASK:

02.03 *Develop an occupation-based intervention plan by selecting intervention strategies and approaches consistent with prioritized needs and best practice in order to facilitate client outcomes.*

Knowledge of:

02.03.01	Activity analysis methods related to client roles, habits and routines, and current abilities
02.03.02	Environments and contexts that maximize participation within areas of occupation
02.03.03	Components of an intervention plan
02.03.04	Methods and techniques for promoting carry-over of intervention within the transitional environment, home, work, school, or community
02.03.05	Life skills relevant to culture, roles, habits, and routines, and current abilities (e.g., home management, social skills, vocational skills)
02.03.06	Frequency and duration of intervention needed to reach goals based on expected outcomes

TASK:

02.04 *Determine the need for referral to other professionals or services using evaluation results in order to facilitate comprehensive, quality care.*

Knowledge of:

02.04.01   Referral sources and processes

02.04.02   Roles and contributions of other service providers

02.04.03   Community resources, funding, reimbursement, and/or payment source

DOMAIN

03   SELECT AND IMPLEMENT EVIDENCE-BASED INTERVENTIONS TO SUPPORT PARTICIPATION IN AREAS OF OCCUPATION (e.g., ADL, education, work, play, leisure, social participation) THROUGHOUT THE CONTINUUM OF CARE

TASK:

03.01 *Use critical reasoning to select and implement interventions and approaches consistent with general medical, neurological, and musculoskeletal conditions and client needs in order to achieve functional outcomes within areas of occupation*

Knowledge of:

03.01.01   Impact of general medical, neurological, and musculoskeletal conditions on areas of occupation (e.g., ADL, work, leisure, social participation, education, play)

03.01.02   Activities to enhance performance within areas of occupation

03.01.03   Compensatory strategies and techniques for minimizing the impact of disease process and/or condition on occupational performance (e.g., joint protection, work simplification, and energy conservation, occupational modification)

03.01.04   Biomechanical strategies and techniques related to body functions and structures (e.g., ROM and strengthening exercises, joint mobilization, wound care, edema control principles and techniques)

03.01.05   Remedial and preventive strategies and techniques specific to general medical conditions (e.g., scar management, pressure-relief techniques, positioning, infection control, standard precautions) for developing or restoring a skill or ability

03.01.06   Facilitation and handling principles and techniques for improving functional performance consistent with general medical, neurological, and/or musculoskeletal conditions

03.01.07   Safe and effective application of superficial and deep thermal, mechanical, and electrotherapeutic physical agent modalities as an adjunct to participation in an activity

03.01.08   Methods for selecting, designing, fabricating splints and/or modifying splints and orthotic devices consistent with general medical, neurological, and/or musculoskeletal conditions

03.01.09	Methods for selecting, designing, fabricating and/or modifying adaptive equipment or assistive devices consistent with general medical, neurological, and/or musculoskeletal conditions
03.01.10	Interventions for facilitating chewing and swallowing specific to general medical conditions
03.01.11	Positioning and physical transfer techniques consistent with activity demands, client skills, and abilities
03.01.12	Neurobehavioral approaches to skill development (e.g., visual scanning, hand-over-hand techniques, visual cueing, verbal prompting) consistent with general medical, neurological, and/or musculoskeletal conditions

TASK:

03.02 *Use critical reasoning to select and implement interventions and approaches consistent with developmental level, pediatric conditions, and/or congenital anomalies and client needs in order to achieve functional outcomes within areas of occupation.*

Knowledge of:

03.02.01	Impact of developmental level, pediatric conditions, and/or congenital anomalies on areas of occupation (e.g., ADL, education, leisure, play, social participation)
03.02.02	Normal development for task accomplishment
03.02.03	Facilitation and handling principles and techniques consistent with developmental level, pediatric conditions, and/or congenital anomalies
03.02.04	Activities to promote development in areas of occupation
03.02.05	Factors that impact visual and perceptual skill development
03.02.06	Sensory integration and sensory modulation principles and techniques
03.02.07	Remedial, compensatory, and preventive techniques specific to developmental level, pediatric conditions, and/or congenital anomalies (e.g., positioning, standard precautions)
03.02.08	Methods for selecting, designing, fabricating splints and/or modifying splints and orthotic devices based on developmental level, pediatric conditions, and/or congenital anomalies
03.02.09	Methods for selecting, designing, fabricating and/or modifying adaptive equipment or assistive devices based on developmental level, pediatric conditions, and/or congenital anomalies
03.02.10	Behavior management principles and techniques appropriate to developmental level
03.02.11	Interventions for facilitating chewing and swallowing specific to developmental level, pediatric conditions, and/or congenital anomalies
03.02.12	Positioning and physical transfer techniques consistent with developmental level and activity demands
03.02.13	Neurobehavioral approaches to skill acquisition consistent with developmental level, pediatric conditions, and/or congenital anomalies (e.g., visual scanning, hand-over-hand techniques, visual cueing, verbal prompting)
03.02.14	Prevocational and vocational exploration processes and procedures

TASK:

03.03 *Use critical reasoning to select and implement interventions and approaches consistent with psychosocial and cognitive abilities, and client needs in order to facilitate outcomes within areas of occupation.*

Knowledge of:

03.03.01	Impact of psychosocial and cognitive abilities on areas of occupation (ADL, work, leisure, social participation)
03.03.02	Methods and techniques for facilitating groups appropriate to participants' psychosocial and cognitive abilities
03.03.03	Activities for enhancing skills within areas of occupation
03.03.04	Methods and techniques for responding in a therapeutic manner to the needs of a client and/or caregiver during psychosocial interventions
03.03.05	Intervention strategies appropriate for psychosocial and cognitive models of practice (e.g., coping skills, stress management, biofeedback, relaxation, cognitive behavioral therapy)
03.03.06	Remedial, compensatory, and preventive techniques consistent with psychosocial and cognitive behavioral status (e.g., problem-solving worksheets, medication management strategies, memory aids, falls prevention)
03.03.07	Methods for selecting, designing, fabricating and/or modifying adaptive equipment or assistive devices consistent with psychosocial and/or cognitive abilities

TASK:

03.04 *Maximize accessibility to and mobility within a client's contexts by identifying and recommending environmental modifications in order to optimize occupational performance and/or enhance quality of life*

Knowledge of:

03.04.01	Principles and methods for environmental modification within contexts (e.g., transitional environments, home, work, school, community)
03.04.02	Accessibility concerns and barriers (e.g., ADA guidelines)
03.04.03	Community transportation alternatives
03.04.04	Types and functions of, and indications and contraindications for seating and mobility systems, durable medical equipment, environmental modifications, and/or assistive technology
03.04.05	Processes and procedures for assessing seating, mobility, assistive technology, and environmental modification needs
03.04.06	Methods for teaching individuals about the safe use and proper care of seating and mobility systems, durable medical equipment, and assistive technology within a variety of contexts
03.04.07	Collaboration strategies for communicating with the client and relevant others (e.g., family, team members, employers, vendors, payors) to acquire and use seating and mobility systems, durable medical equipments and/or assistive technology
03.04.08	Ergonomic principles and universal design
03.04.09	Methods for adapting the home and/or community environment

TASK:

03.05 *Modify interventions based on the client's needs and responses in order to promote occupational performance.*

Knowledge of:

03.05.01   Physical, psychological, and social responses requiring modification of the intervention

03.05.02   Methods for adjusting intervention techniques in response to variances from anticipated outcomes

03.05.03   Methods for adapting the intervention environment based on medical status and behavioral responses that maximize participation within areas of occupation

03.05.04   Methods for grading an intervention activity based on expected progress and/or unexpected physical responses

03.05.05   Methods for responding appropriately to unexpected occurrences during intervention

TASK:

03.06 *Apply the principles of health promotion, wellness, prevention and/or educational programming based on client and community needs in order to provide information or serve as a resource consultant for occupation based program activities.*

Knowledge of:

03.06.01   Consultation and advocacy principles related to health promotion, wellness, prevention and/or educational programming for at-risk populations

03.06.02   Methods for identifying service needs for at-risk populations

DOMAIN

04   UPHOLD PROFESSIONAL STANDARDS AND RESPONSIBILITIES TO PROMOTE QUALITY IN PRACTICE

TASK:

04.01 *Maintain ongoing competence by participating in professional development activities and appraising evidence-based literature using critical reasoning skills in order to provide effective services and promote quality care.*

Knowledge of:

04.01.01   Professional development activities

04.01.02   NBCOT certification renewal policies

04.01.03   Validity and reliability concepts

04.01.04   Methods for analyzing data and interpreting data in literature

TASK:

04.02 *Uphold professional standards by participating in continuous quality improvement activities and complying with safety regulations, laws, ethical codes, facility policies and procedures, and guidelines governing OT practice in order to protect the public interest.*

Knowledge of:

04.02.01	Policies, procedures, and guidelines related to service provision
04.02.02	Ethical decision-making
04.02.03	NBCOT code of conduct
04.02.04	Client confidentiality regulations (e.g., HIPAA)
04.02.05	State and federal laws governing OT practice
04.02.06	Methods for incorporating federally mandated guidelines into intervention plans
04.02.07	Safety procedures and risk management techniques
04.02.08	Accrediting bodies and their requirements
04.02.09	Standards/scope of practice for OT
04.02.10	Quality improvement processes and procedures (includes program evaluation and outcomes measures)

TASK:

04.03 *Document occupational therapy services and outcomes using established guidelines in order to verify accountability and to meet the requirements of practice settings, accrediting bodies, regulatory agencies and/or funding sources.*

Knowledge of:

04.03.01	Methods and purposes for documentation
04.03.02	Reimbursement systems and regulatory requirements for documentation

TASK:

04.04 *Articulate how occupational therapy contributes to beneficial outcomes for clients and relevant others based on evidence in order to promote quality care.*

Knowledge of:

04.04.01	Roles and responsibilities of certified OT practitioners
04.04.02	Effective communication methods and strategies

TASK:

04.05 *Supervise assistants, paraprofessionals, students, and volunteers in accordance with professional guidelines and applicable regulations in order to support the delivery of appropriate occupational therapy services.*

Knowledge of:

04.05.01	OTR and COTA role delineation
04.05.02	Clinical fieldwork education
04.05.03	Regulatory requirements and professional standards for supervision